Parents' Guide to Speech and Deafness

Parents' Guide
to
Speech and Deafness

By

Donald R. Calvert

Director, Central Institute for the Deaf
Professor of Audiology, Washington University

Alexander Graham Bell Association for the Deaf
Washington, D.C.

The Alexander Graham Bell Association for the Deaf, Inc.
3417 Volta Place, N.W., Washington, D.C. 20007, U.S.A.

Library of Congress Catalogue Card Number 84-070988
ISBN 0-88200-155-8

Dedicated to
Beth, Howard, Clare, Hajime, Cinde, and Richard:
parents of hearing-impaired children who
inspired this book in the first place,
and then offered valuable suggestions
for improving the manuscript.

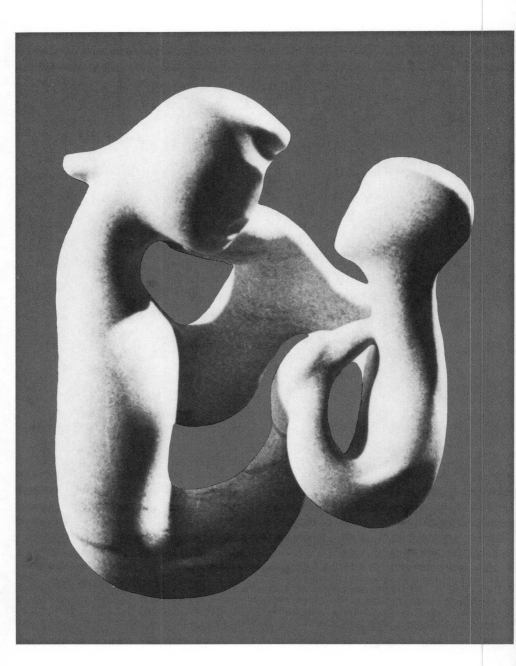

Sculpture Legend

The white marble sculpture, "Learners," that stands in the entry of the Central Institute School was created by Hillis Arnold of St. Louis, recalling his mother as his first teacher. It symbolizes the personal intimacy of teaching/learning speech, and its title reflects the perpetual learning about speech by both the children involved and by the adults, be they teachers, parents, or anyone in any way who lends support to this worthy endeavor.

Contents

List of Tables

List of Figures

Introduction

Hearing-impaired children <u>can</u> learn to talk! This statement has been true for at least four hundred and fifty years since a Spanish monk first taught children to speak in order to say catechisms. **Not all hearing-impaired children <u>do</u> learn to talk!** That statement is as true today as it was in the sixteenth century. These related facts suggest the questions that parents most often ask and that professionals have a very hard time answering:

Will *my* child be able to learn to talk? If so, how *good* will the speech be?

No one can really answer those questions for the parents of a hearing-impaired baby. In fact, parents should be wary of those who do so with absolute confidence, whether their answers are positive or negative. We're learning about some things that help predict how well hearing-impaired children might eventually learn to talk—the varying factors that people in research measure and relate to later performance. We don't know all these varying factors or how to measure them yet, but we do know some of them.

That's what this book is about—what helps hearing-impaired children learn to talk. One thing we know from experience is that parents and other family members can help a lot. In fact, they are **essential** to the team effort for most children. This book was prepared as a guide to parents who want their hearing-impaired children to learn to talk and who want to be included in the act of teaching.

It is common in schools to have teachers' guides to textbooks or to courses. This *Parents' Guide to Speech and Deafness* recognizes the unusual importance of family members and their vital part in the special task of

1

teaching hearing-impaired children to talk. It will not prepare you to be a classroom teacher of hearing-impaired children, but it does consider you as an active participant in the teaching process.

This *Parents' Guide* is written to accompany the textbook *Speech and Deafness.* * The original text has been in use by teachers since 1975 and was revised in 1983. It was designed to help prepare student-teachers, and to be used as a reference for working teachers, speech pathologists and audiologists. This *Guide* is designed for parents who may or may not wish to read the textbook. References to pages in the revised 1983 edition of the book are included in bracketed bold type within the text of this *Guide* for those who wish to study further. Teachers, speech pathologists, audiologists, or administrators may recommend the *Guide* as reading to help parents understand what is happening in the clinic or classroom, and what they can do at home. Some parents may want to read it just to know more about speech or to find out how they can "get into the act."

Although prepared especially for parents, this *Guide* may also be helpful to regular classroom teachers or speech pathologists, prepared for working with normal-hearing children, who may now find they have responsibility for one or more hearing-impaired children in their classroom or clinic caseload. For such professionals, this *Guide* can be both an introduction to the subject and a useful reference to appropriate sections of *Speech and Deafness* which they may wish to read in more detail.

This *Guide* is organized around several questions that parents commonly ask, *and some questions that parents usually don't ask but should ask.* It begins with what we understand about the influence of impaired hearing on learning and producing speech, which is really the nature of the problem. The first chapter includes some ideas that may help you explain to your friends and family the unusual sound of your child's speech. The second chapter introduces the ways we measure and describe hearing in order to observe important differences among children and take advantage of whatever hearing they may have left. This may help you with the terms and graphs used by audiologists and teachers. Chapter 3 describes how a hearing aid works, what it can do for speech, and what it can't do for speech. The next chapter gets to some practical suggestions you might use to help your child take full advantage of whatever hearing is still available to him, especially in learning and producing speech.

Chapter 5 reviews common approaches for teaching speech to hearing-impaired children used in schools and clinics. This is a good starting point for you to ask some questions and learn about your child's own school program. The last chapter summarizes some ideas, suggested by both parents and teachers, to aid family members to share in helping hearing-impaired

---

*Calvert, Donald R. and Silverman, S. Richard, *Speech & Deafness,* Revised Edition, Washington, D.C.: Alexander Graham Bell Association for the Deaf, 1983.

children to learn and use speech effectively. Some of these may be useful for you, and you will probably find some suggestions of your own to add to them. If you do, I would appreciate your suggestions for possible inclusion in future revisions of this *Guide*.

Donald R. Calvert, Ph.D.
Central Institute for the Deaf
818 South Euclid Avenue
St. Louis, Missouri 63110

CHAPTER I

Why Don't Hearing-Impaired Children Learn to Talk Naturally?*

Long ago people believed that deaf children did not talk because their speech organs—the tongue, lips, and palate—were defective. Some thought there was a single place in the brain that controlled both hearing and speech, and that children who didn't hear didn't talk because that place was injured. It took a long time to understand that hearing is the *primary sense* necessary for learning and controlling speech. When hearing is impaired, impaired speech will result. Probably this fact was first noticed when people observed that those who were losing their hearing as they grew older also began to have poorer speech. Table 1 includes some common observations that relate speech to hearing impairment.

WHAT IS IT LIKE TO TRY TO TALK WITHOUT HEARING?

You cannot have exactly the same feeling that your hearing-impaired child does unless you have a severe hearing loss yourself. Since over 90 per-

---

*Bold face page references in text, table and figures are to: Calvert, Donald R. and Silverman, S. Richard, *Speech and Deafness,* Revised edition, Washington, DC: Alexander Graham Bell Association for the Deaf, 1983.

For People Losing Their Hearing	For People Born With Impaired Hearing
1. As a person born with normal hearing loses hearing, speech begins to deteriorate.	A child born with severe hearing impairment does not acquire speech naturally or adequately. **[pp. 66–67]**
2. The greater the hearing loss becomes, the greater the deterioration of the speech.	The greater the hearing impairment, the poorer the child's speech and the harder it is for him to acquire or develop it.
3. As hearing loss becomes more severe, changes in speech occur first in articulation, and then in voice quality and finally in speech rhythm.	A child with mild-to-moderate hearing impairment has deviations in articulation. With severe hearing impairment, deviations will also occur in voice quality and speech rhythm.

Table 1. Common observations that relate speech to hearing impairment.

cent of the parents of deaf children have normal hearing, this section is addressed to those parents. There are a few ways to help you understand what it might be like to talk without hearing. You may remember being in a very noisy place where you literally could not hear yourself talk. Do you also recall that you shouted in order to hear what you were saying? That's how important hearing is. Once we have learned to talk, we continue to depend upon our hearing to "monitor" our speech, that is, to tell us whether we produced the intended sounds clearly and loud enough **[pp. 50, 121]**. If you can arrange it, have an audiologist or a teacher deliver loud steady noise to you through earphones. Now, talk to someone and notice that you are more aware of the movement of your tongue and lips, especially when the outside noise is loud enough so that you cannot hear yourself talk. You are also probably talking too loud for others as you try to raise your voice so that you can hear yourself.

A similar experience is to talk without using your voice. Don't whisper, because even that gives "feedback" that you can hear and that helps you monitor your own speech. Notice that you are now also more aware of the movement of your tongue and lips than when you could hear your voice normally. Say the word "tooth" without voice and feel where the tongue touches.

Here is another experiment you can do that will give you a feel for what it is like to write without vision—a situation that is a little like talking without hearing. Follow the directions carefully, taking them one step at a time. It won't do any good just to read the instructions:

First, get a pencil and a sheet of paper. Place them in front of you as you sit at a table or desk. Clear everything off around you so that nothing will get in your way. Now pick up the pencil and just get ready to write near the top of the page in handwriting script the phrase "excellent living accommodations." But just before you begin writing, close your eyes tightly so that you cannot see at all. Don't peek!

How did you do? Did you cross the *x* and both letters *t*? Did you dot the three letters *i*? Are the spaces between the words too large or too small? Did you write uphill or downhill? Did you write larger or smaller than ususal? Could anyone read your writing? Is that the way you usually write?

Now let's see what can be learned from this exercise:

1. First of all, you **did** write the phrase even though you couldn't see the paper. You did not have available the *primary* sense for controlling your writing—seeing. But you could feel something as you wrote. You could feel the movement of your hand and fingers following the familiar shapes of the letters of the alphabet. You used *secondary* senses to monitor writing—the senses of touch and muscle movement. These are called the "tactile" and the "kinesthetic" senses. **[pp. 24–25]** *A child who cannot hear depends upon these secondary senses to feel how he is speaking.*

2. Although the secondary senses gave you some feedback from the action of writing, they were not accurate enough for you to write as well as usual. Even if you practiced again and again, writing with your eyes closed would not be the same as writing with your eyes open. *The speech of a child who does not hear will not sound the same as a child who has normal hearing.*

Now let's change the experiment a little to emphasize another point. *Place a pencil and a sheet of paper in front of you as you sit at a table or desk. Pick up the pencil and prepare to write the same phrase, "excellent living accommodations," near the top of the paper. But this time, cheat a little. Squint your eyes so that you can't see normally, but enough that you can peek at what you are writing. Now write.*

How did you do this time? Why was it so much easier and the result so much better? Does using some of the primary monitoring sense help handwriting? What we can learn from this experiment is obvious.

3. A little bit of the primary sense that monitors writing can make a big improvement, and make it much easier to write. There is a somewhat similar result with hearing and speech. *If even a little hearing can be used to monitor a child's speech, the speech will be better and it will be easier for the child to speak.* **[pp. 65–66]**

Now go back and try the experiment the first way, with your eyes closed tightly. Then ask yourself, *Is a hearing aid that is in good working order important for a child who has a little bit of usable hearing?* You bet it is!

WILL THE SPEECH OF HEARING-IMPAIRED CHILDREN GRADUALLY GET BETTER AND BETTER?

We have to answer that by saying "yes and no." That is not just avoiding the question. From experience, teachers notice some typical periods of improvement and leveling off in speech development. Children with normal hearing gradually improve their speaking ability until they have mastered all the speech sounds, usually by age seven to nine years. Their speech stays at about that level for most of their lives unless they make a special effort to improve diction or practice public speaking.

For children with severe or profound hearing impairment, it is common to see slow progress at first. It depends, of course, on special instruction. Then their speech seems to get a lot better at about age six or seven years as they have learned to produce most of the speech sounds, when they have a lot of words they can use, and after they have learned the simple language structures (grammar) used by children at that age. But hearing-impaired children are not just learning the mechanics of speech. They are learning to speak the English language. Their vocabulary grows with many new words that are more difficult to pronounce. In addition, the grammatical structures get more difficult and more varied as a child continues to learn language. Children often have to stop to think about how a sentence should be said—what words to use, what order the words should be in, whether a verb should be past or present tense, whether a noun is plural or singular.

Since those of us with normal hearing learned all this through our ears, we can formulate speech in a split-second and don't have to think about it. As hearing-impaired children *do* think about it while they are talking, their speech will be slowed down and may become choppy so that the natural flow of speech rhythm will be interrupted. **[p. 43]** *When hearing-impaired children are learning and using a lot of new language, their speech may seem harder to understand.*

It is also true that when children are very young we often know just what they are going to talk about so that it is easy to understand their speech, however imprecise it may be. As they grow older and want to talk about a variety of things we may not be aware of, their speech will naturally seem harder to understand.

So, sometimes during the elementary years you might be disappointed about what seems to be lack of speech progress. However, your child is really making progress as he learns our difficult English language and practices using it until most phrases become automatic. *Learning to use language is one of the most difficult tasks for hearing-impaired children, and their ability to use language influences their speech directly.* Once they have mastered the structures and rules of English and can use them automatically, their speech is likely to improve again and be even better than before.

Another thing we've observed is that some speech sounds seem especially hard for hearing-impaired children to *maintain* as they grow older. **[pp. 112–113]** That is, even though certain sounds have been "learned" in school, and children can produce the sounds alone and in words when they are practicing them, they don't seem to *use* them when they talk in conversation. The **s** sound is one of these; the **sh** and the **ch** are others. **[pp. 162– 164]** The use of these sounds never seems to improve. That is because hearing-impaired children cannot *monitor* them well. **[pp. 193–200]** The **s** sound has high-pitched energy that may not be reproduced by a typical hearing aid so that this sound may not be monitored at all through the child's primary sense for monitoring speech—hearing. **[p. 121]** The **s** does not have a very definite tongue position or sensation of touching the teeth or the inside of the mouth, either, so that it is not well monitored by the secondary senses—the tactile and kinesthetic senses. Try making the words "tea" and "sea" *without any sound* and feel how much stronger tactile-kinesthetic monitoring is for the **t** sound compared to the **s** sound.

Hearing-impaired children probably do not forget to produce the **s** sound in conversation, but they can't monitor it well enough to be sure that we hear it. *Hearing-impaired persons will probably need help and reminders about some speech sounds throughout their life.* **[pp. 174–176]**

WHY DON'T HEARING-IMPAIRED CHILDREN LEARN TO TALK NATURALLY?

It is not really possible for those of us with normal hearing to remember how we learned to speak our language. Psychologists and linguists (specialists in language) have studied this by observing children as they grow up. A relatively new specialty called "psycho-linguistics" is making careful observations of the *interactions* between children and their parents to see what are the necessary factors to learn a language. **[pp. 124–125]** We are beginning to understand the necessary learning process for children with normal hearing and this helps us to understand why hearing-impaired children don't learn to talk naturally.

Here are some general observations that help answer the question that is the title of this chapter. "Why Don't Hearing-Impaired Children Learn to Talk Naturally?"

   1. Children need to experience *many* examples of each word or unit of speech in order to have models to imitate and remember. Hearing-impaired children cannot receive nearly as many examples of words or language as children with normal hearing.

2. Children need *clear* examples of speech in order to imitate it accurately. The few examples that hearing-impaired children receive are likely to be distorted, indistinct, and even confusing.

3. Children need to be able to hear how their own speech sounds in order to *compare* it directly to the examples they have heard as others speak. Hearing-impaired children are not able to monitor their speech entirely through their hearing, nor can they compare their own speech directly with that of others through hearing.

4. Children need to hear or see many examples of spoken *language* in order to associate words with meaning and to understand grammar. Hearing-impaired children will not develop understanding and use of English naturally. A child's ability to use *language* influences how well he understands speech.

These are very general observations, but when we want to apply them to a particular child, we need to know what that child is capable of hearing. It is very clear that whatever hearing capacity a "hearing-impaired child" has, it is important for him in learning and producing speech. The opportunity for each child to make the best use of hearing begins with the measurement and description of hearing. This is part of the subject matter of the field called "audiology." The next chapter reviews some aspects of audiology that are useful for parents.

CHAPTER II

Should You Say "Deaf" or "Hearing Impaired"?*

These words do *not* mean the same thing. It is important to know how to use them because the words we use have a lot to do with how we think, and how we think about children influences what we do for them.

For example, some people still use the old terms "deaf and dumb" or "deaf mute." Both phrases suggest that hearing-impaired children do not talk. We know that some don't talk, but that many do. It is likely that most people don't know any better than to use those terms for all hearing-impaired children, and it is up to all of us to help set them straight. *But, suppose we treated all hearing-impaired children as "deaf and dumb," as if they could not talk.* Then we would *not try* to teach them to talk because that would be a waste of time. If we did not try to teach them to talk, and if they did not learn on their own because of the reasons we noted in the first chapter, they would not learn to talk. Then we might say, "See, deaf and dumb children don't talk." That is called a *self-fulfilling prophecy*—a prediction that came true because we made it come true.

The word "deaf" brings to mind some negative thoughts about people. What is more important, the word "deaf" was used for many years to mean *complete absence* of hearing. At one time it was applied to *all* children who

---

*Page references in boldface within text refer to: Calvert, Donald R. and Silverman, S. Richard *Speech and Deafness,* Revised Edition, Washington, DC: Alexander Graham Bell Association for the Deaf, 1983.

10

were enrolled in special schools, then called "asylums" for deaf children. That was at a time when hearing was not tested, measured and described as it is today. Of course, at that time, it made no difference whether or not a child's hearing was tested because that was before electronic hearing aids were available to take full advantage of usable hearing. *The important thing is that the word "deaf" was regularly applied to all the children in special schools and institutions, regardless of their level of hearing.*

"Deaf" children were not expected to learn or accomplish very much in many of our early schools. It didn't make any difference how much usable hearing any of the children had because it was not used, in any case. They were considered as "deaf children" and deaf children were supposed to be limited in what they could learn. Because they were *treated* that way, they did *not* learn very much. Another self-fulfilling prophecy!

But then mechanical hearing aids and later electronic hearing aids began to be used in a few schools for deaf children, and some children began to improve in their speech and lipreading when they wore these new amplifiers. The children with more hearing than others began to learn and achieve more, not as well as children with normal hearing, but much better than was *expected* of "deaf" children. Suddenly it became important to measure children's hearing and to treat them individually, according to the amount of hearing *each* child had. Calling all hearing-impaired children "deaf" didn't seem to fit any more.

But ideas change very slowly. Although the first electric-powered hearing aids were available about the year 1900, they were not used with very many deaf children until the 1920s or 1930s, and then only in a few schools. It was not until around 1950 that research studies on hearing-impaired children convincingly demonstrated improvement in understanding speech when amplification and auditory training were used in schools. Even though there were rapid advances in hearing aids with the invention of transistors and miniature printed circuits, many schools thought the new hearing aids were not for "deaf" children. To their teachers, "deaf" still meant "without any usable hearing," and it seemed foolish to use the expensive and bothersome instruments for these children. The use of this older word, "deaf," when applied to all hearing-impaired children in the schools, was influencing what was being done for them.

The term "hearing-impaired" began to be applied to all children who did not have normal hearing, in order to recognize the range of critical differences in hearing ability among children. It included children with a mild-to-moderate impairment (sometimes called "hard-of-hearing"), and those with more severe and even profound hearing impairment. It seemed more accurate to use the term "hearing impaired" for the entire group of children and to restrict the word "deaf" only to those who had almost no usable hearing at all. As hearing aids have been getting more and more powerful, the group of hearing-impaired children requiring the label "deaf" has been getting smaller and smaller. Use of the term "hearing *loss*" should be limited to impairment that has happened or increased after the child was born. Figure 1 represents graphically the uses of *hearing impaired* and *deaf* for children who do not have normal hearing.

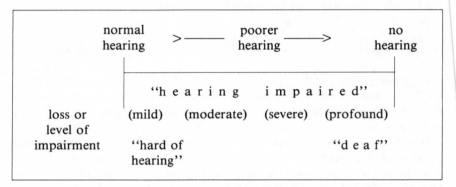

Figure 1. Terms used to describe conditions of hearing.

HOW IS IT POSSIBLE TO USE LIMITED HEARING TO TEACH SPEECH?

Even when a child's hearing is severely impaired, it may still be used to teach speech for the following reasons. **[pp. 67–68]**

1. Hearing impairment is seldom total. Complete deafness is rare and most hearing-impaired children have a useful remnant of hearing that can be demonstrated by measurement.

2. Not all of the sounds of speech need be heard for speech to be useful. Some features of speech, such as its rhythm, are transmitted simply by the presence or absence of sound or by low-pitched sound, and even very severely hearing-impaired children can learn to use these.

3. Hearing aids and classroom amplifiers can make up for some hearing impairment, particularly by making speech sounds audible—the children's own speech and that of others. Great progress has been made in designing powerful, wearable hearing aids, and continued progress is likely.

4. Parents and teachers can work together to see that children make the best possible use of hearing aids all day and every day. They can follow a program of medical and audiological preventive care, making sure hearing aids are always working well and not constantly "in the shop" for repair.

5. Parents and teachers can work together to see that children receive the sounds of speech clearly through their hearing aids, both during activities at home and through special instruction at school.

All of this suggests that a lot of direct action and hard work are necessary in order to use hearing to develop, encourage and maintain speech. *Just putting a hearing aid on won't do it!* It involves much more work and some of that is described in the other chapters of this book. The task right now is to understand more about hearing and how it is measured.

WHAT SHOULD YOU KNOW ABOUT AN AUDIOGRAM?

An audiogram can tell a lot but it doesn't tell you everything about hearing. The "audiogram" is a chart on which an "audiologist," a specialist in hearing, records responses to a hearing test. **[pp. 68–71]** In a hearing test, tones are delivered to either ear through the earphones of an "audiometer," an instrument to measure hearing. When the softest level of a tone is given at which the listener can just detect the tone and respond, that level is recorded on the audiogram as the listener's *hearing-threshold* level. Sometimes it is called simply the "hearing level" or the "threshold level." People with "normal hearing" do not hear tones of different pitches equally well. The audiometer and the audiogram adjust for this normal variation and designate the average threshold level for normal listeners as a 0 (zero) level for each of the tones of different pitches. The remainder of the audiogram compares the threshold responses of a particular person to normal hearing. Use the audiogram form in Figure 2 as an example.

The vertical direction of the form shows differences in *intensity*, the physical measure that is related to *loudness*. As you go down the graph, the numbers get larger and the sounds become stronger. The sound level of 20 decibels* is very soft, like rustling leaves. The level of 120 decibels would be extremely loud to a normal ear, similar to the noise near a jet airplane engine. However this might be merely a very soft sound, very near threshold level for some profoundly deaf listeners.

The horizontal direction of the form shows differences in *frequency*, the physical measure that is related to the *pitch* we hear. As you go across the graph, the numbers get larger and the sounds become higher in pitch. A tone of 125 Hertz** has a low frequency, about like a male bass voice. An 8000 Hertz tone has a high frequency we would hear as very high-pitched, like a thin, high whistle.

These two dimensions of sound on the audiogram reflect the range of hearing of the normal ear—from sounds that can barely be heard to those that are too loud to tolerate, and from sounds that have the lowest pitch to those that have the highest pitch the ear can hear. Many audiometers are not

---

*Intensity changes are measured in Bels, named for Alexander Graham Bell, and one-tenth of a Bel is a "decibel," abbreviated *dB*.

**Frequency levels, the number of sound vibration cycles in a second, are called "Hertz," after Heinrich Hertz, a nineteenth century German physicist, and abbreviated *Hz*.

powerful enough to test children with severe-to-profound hearing levels and you may need to find a hearing clinic with specially designed audiometers that reach to appropriate levels for your child. Some children can hear tones as high as 20,000 Hertz, and special equipment that reaches that high in frequency is available in only a few hearing clinics.

When a listener's threshold level is reached for the tone being tested, the audiologist marks the audiogram form at the intersection of vertical and horizontal lines that correspond to the frequency and intensity of the tone. **[pp. 69–70]** It is customary to use a circle (○) to mark responses for the right ear and an X mark for the left ear. Look at Figure 2, for example,

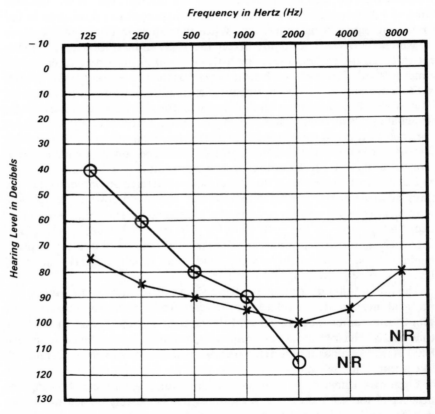

Figure 2. *A pure-tone audiogram form with hearing levels and hearing curves for the right ear (○) and left ear (X) of a person with severe-to-profound hearing level. NR indicates that no response was given to a tone at maximum intensity output of the audiometer.*

where the threshold of a 500-Hertz tone for the right ear is marked at 80 decibels. The threshold of a 2000-Hertz tone for the left ear is marked at 100 decibels.

All these marks on the audiogram for each of seven tones in two ears make it hard to talk about hearing in simple terms. Audiologists do several things to simplify this information. First, the hearing-threshold levels for tones on each ear are connected by a line to form an *audiometric curve.* Second, the hearing-threshold levels for each ear are commonly referred to by a *single decibel level.* **[p. 71]** This is usually the average level of 500 Hertz, 1000 Hertz, and 2000 Hertz, because these three frequencies are considered most important for hearing speech. They are sometimes called the "speech frequencies." In Figure 2, the average for the left ear is 95 decibels (90 + 95 + 100 divided by 3). The third simplification is to refer only to the *better ear* when talking about a child's hearing because if hearing in the two ears is very different, the child is likely to respond to speech primarily in the better of the two ears. In Figure 2, the two ears of the hearing-impaired child happen to have the very same speech frequency average, even though the ears are very different. An audiologist might refer to this child simply as having a 95-decibel hearing level. What would your child's hearing level be for each ear? For the better ear?

. Large population studies use this "better-ear average" to report hearing-threshold levels among hearing-impaired children. For example, a recent report of hearing levels in the United States among children who were enrolled in special schools and classes for hearing-impaired children showed these proportions:

Under 40 decibels .... 10 percent
41 to 55 decibels................................. 9 percent
56 to 70 decibels................................. 13 percent
71 to 90 decibels................................. 25 percent
91 decibels and above .... 43 percent

Another use of the better-ear speech-frequency averages is in relating hearing-threshold levels to expected differences in speech and language for children. Table 2 relates some commonly grouped hearing levels to speech and language expectations. Into which of these groups would your child fit?

Of course the audiologist will also want to find out whether a child's hearing level is influenced by a *conductive hearing loss* involving the middle portion of the ear. If this is the case, audiologists and physicians have tests that help decide whether any medical treatment or even an operation might improve hearing. But still other test information is important, especially for fitting hearing aids. **[pp. 75–77]** Audiologists who are competent to test severely or profoundly hearing-impaired children may report much more information on an audiogram form than just thresholds, especially for older children. **[p. 88]**

Hearing-Threshold Levels	Speech and Language Expectations
– 10 to 20 decibels (normal hearing)	No related speech or language deviations.
20 to 35 decibels (mild hearing impairment)	No related speech deviations. Language may be slower in developing.
35 to 55 decibels (mild-to-moderate hearing impairment)	Some defects of articulation. Speech and language may be slower in developing.
55 to 70 decibels (moderate hearing impairment)	Abnormalities of articulation and voice. Vocabulary may be deficient.
70 to 90 decibels (severe hearing impairment)	Articulation and voice quality likely to be abnormal. Syntax and other aspects of language may be deficient. Will need to be taught to speak.
90 decibels or poorer (severe-to-profound hearing impairment)	Speech rhythm, voice and articulation likely to be abnormal. Speech and language must be developed with careful and extensive training. Supplements to the auditory channel will be helpful.
100 decibels or poorer (profound hearing impairment)	The auditory channel is often helpful, but will need use of non-auditory channels for speech development.

Table 2. Hearing levels (better ear average) related to speech and language learning by children, and expected deviations in speech and language.

CAN SOUND EVER BE TOO LOUD FOR A "DEAF" CHILD?

A common misunderstanding about "deaf" children is that they are never bothered by loud noises. This popular belief resulted in training hearing-impaired people to work around noisy machinery, such as printing presses. This old mistaken notion was caused by using the word "deaf" to mean "no hearing." But many hearing-impaired children are sensitive to loud sounds, and the small amount of usable hearing they have may be damaged if the ear is exposed to loud noise for long periods of time. Many hearing-impaired children feel discomfort or even pain when noise is extremely loud, just as children or adults with normal hearing would.

An audiologist can test hearing-impaired children for their *tolerance* to loud noises. This is commonly done by gradually increasing the level of tones or bands of noise at different frequencies until the child reports that the sound is too loud. **[pp. 71–73]** Of course, such a test must be done carefully by a skilled audiologist with a powerful audiometer. The results

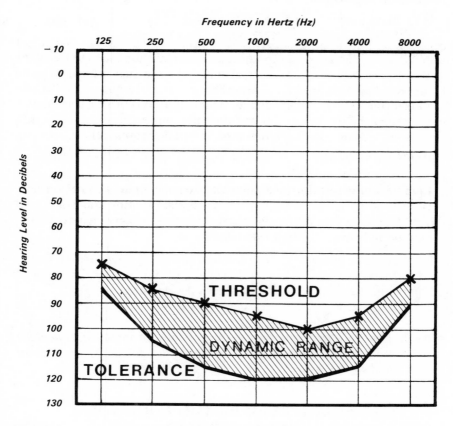

Figure 3. A pure-tone audiogram form with hearing-threshold levels and hearing curve for the left ear (X) of a person with severe-to-profound hearing level, the tolerance level for each frequency measured for the left ear, and the resulting dynamic range of hearing in that ear.

can be placed on the same audiogram form where threshold responses were marked down. Since each ear is likely to be different, it is necessary to use two audiogram forms—one for each ear.

Now the audiologist can show you "dynamic range configuration" audiograms, like that in Figure 3, which include both the threshold curve and the tolerance curve for each ear. You can see the range between the lowest hearing level of soft sounds for just hearing each frequency tested and the level at which the sound is too loud. This range of usable hearing is called the "dynamic range" (tolerance level minus hearing-threshold level = dynamic range). Notice the dynamic range of hearing for the left ear represented by the shaded area on the audiogram of Figure 3. *The dynamic range of normal hearing is very wide* (100 decibels or more), *but for a hearing-impaired child the range may be very small.*

The size of the dynamic range at each frequency is important in the fitting of an appropriate hearing aid. After all, a hearing aid is a device that makes sounds louder, and an inappropriate one could make the sound too loud for a child's tolerance level. It is important that a hearing aid increase the loudness of sound beyond the hearing-threshold level so that a child is able to hear it, but that the aid should not increase the loudness so much that it goes beyond the tolerance level and becomes unpleasant or even painful. *The dynamic range presents a target for the skilled audiologist in selecting an appropriate hearing aid for each of the ears of each child tested.*

Careful measurement of hearing is the first step in helping children use hearing to learn speech. Selection of appropriate hearing aids is the next step and the following chapter is concerned with what hearing aids can and cannot do in helping children learn speech.

CHAPTER III

What Does A Hearing Aid Do For Speech?*

A hearing aid or amplifier is a device that makes sound louder. *It does not make the ear or hearing more normal.* That is an important difference. Even though children may learn to listen better with appropriate amplification, and may learn to make use of parts of the sound to help them understand the speech of others and to produce their own speech, scientists agree that their ears will not be improved. It is believed, however, that if a hearing-impaired child is not stimulated by sound-through-amplification at an early age, the auditory nervous system may not develop as completely as it can. *Do not expect miracles from hearing aids,* but because they are so very important for learning speech, parents should understand how they work and how they should be used.

JUST HOW DOES A HEARING AID MAKE SPEECH SOUND LOUDER?

The simplest form of speech amplification is to "speak up" or move closer to the listener. If there is an older person with hearing loss in your

---

*Bold face page references in the text are to: Calvert, Donald R. and Silverman, S. Richard, *Speech and Deafness,* Revised Edition, Washington, DC: Alexander Graham Bell Association for the Deaf, 1983.

family, you may have already used this tiring kind of speech amplification. **[p. 89]** Long before electronic hearing aids, very young, hearing-impaired children in a few schools were taught on a teacher's lap as she spoke in a strong voice directly into their ears. Early mechanical hearing aids, like ear trumpets, used the principle of the funnel, altering the original sound by collecting sound energy over a large area and presenting it to the ear, concentrated in a smaller area. Such devices raised the intensity of the original sound about 10 to 30 decibels, enough to help a person with a mild hearing impairment.

Electronic amplification uses the principle of substituting a strong new source of sound for the original weaker one, and using the original sound to tailor the pattern of the new sound. **[pp. 89–92]** Sound waves, similar to speech, can be produced by electronic equipment, using a battery or electrical current from a wall socket to push the thin diaphragm of a loud speaker or earphone. This electronically produced sound can be much stronger than is possible for sound produced by a human speaker. Figure 4 illustrates the nature of *electronic* or *electro-acoustic amplification.* **[pp. 90–91]**

Basic electro-acoustic amplification systems consist of the following components:

1. *A microphone* to receive the sound waves of the original speech signal and convert or "transduce" them to a pattern of electrical current.

2. *A source of electrical power,* such as a battery, that produces a strong, steady flow of electrical current.

3. *An amplifying circuit* that brings together the pattern of electrical current from the microphone and the strong steady flow of electrical current from the power source in a transistor-valving action that tailors the pattern of the strong current from the power source.

4. *An earphone* (sometimes called a "receiver") that receives the strong pattern of electrical current and converts or transduces it into a pattern of sound waves that forms a strong speech signal.

5. *Controls* that usually include an "on-off" switch to prohibit or permit the flow of current from the power source, and a volume dial to reduce or increase the flow of current and thus the loudness level from the power source.

Now let's return to the testing of hearing that we began in the last chapter and consider the fitting of hearing aids for each child. Figure 3 in Chapter 2 illustrated the dynamic range of hearing between the hearing-threshold level and the hearing-tolerance level. We said then (see page 18) that the dynamic range for each ear of a child was the target for the audiologist in selecting an appropriate hearing aid.

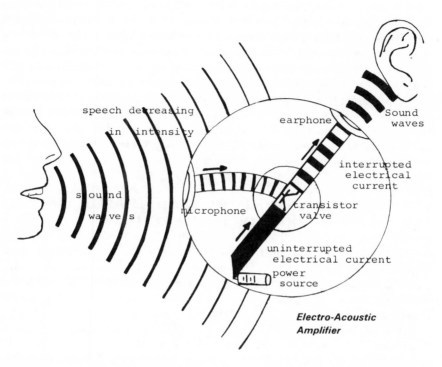

Figure 4. *Diagram to illustrate the principle of electro-acoustic amplification. Speech sound waves from the mouth, too weak to be audible to the distant or impaired ear, are received by a microphone of the electro-acoustic amplifier. Here they are converted to electrical energy and transmitted to transistors in an amplifying circuit. A power source drives a strong, steady electrical current to the transistor where the current is interrupted by the energy pattern from the microphone. The strong electrical current, mirroring the pattern of energy from the microphone, pushes against the diaphragm of a loudspeaker or earphone, creating a strong pattern of sound waves that is received by the ear.*

HOW WELL CAN AN AUDIOLOGIST HIT THE DYNAMIC RANGE TARGET?

That will depend on the size of the dynamic range, the engineering "know how" of the maker of the hearing aid, and the skill of the audiologist. Hearing aids have come a long way recently in the amount of power or "gain" in increasing sound that they can produce, and also in the control or limit they have on loud sounds, called their "maximum power output." Both the *gain* and the *maximum power output* of a hearing aid will be different for each frequency. **[pp. 92–95]** *The maximum power output of a hearing aid should not be at the tolerance level or go beyond the tolerance level for any frequency tested for your child's ears.* By adjusting the maximum power output of a hearing aid for sound at each frequency, the audiologist can see that a powerful hearing aid does not give your child any discomfort from loud sounds. Then, if there is a sudden loud noise, your child will be protected. *The maximum power output of a hearing aid for each tested frequency can be included on the audiogram with some computation by the audiologist or by other hearing aid distributors.*

WHAT DOES A HEARING AID DO FOR THE SOUNDS OF SPEECH?

Once you are sure that the maximum power output of a hearing aid is appropriate to protect your child's ear, you should be interested in finding out what the aid can do for the sounds of speech. **[pp. 78–89]** Of course you will want your child to hear other sounds as well, but we know that hearing *speech* may help him greatly in learning to speak.

Although 500 Hertz, 1000 Hertz, and 2000 Hertz are commonly called "the speech frequencies," the sounds of our speech really range from the low-pitched sounds of 100 Hertz in some vowels to over 8000 Hertz in such consonants as **s** and **sh**. The more of this range we can hear, the easier it is to understand speech. *The more of this range the child can hear, the easier it should be for him to learn to speak.*

Speech also has a range of changes in loudness from moment to moment. From such loud vowels as the **aw** in *law,* to the very soft consonants such as the **f** in *fin* or the **th** in *thin,* there is a range of nearly 30 decibels **[p. 24]**. In a word like *thaw,* the ear needs to be able to hear sounds over this entire range of loudness. The more of this range we can hear, the easier it is to understand speech. *The more of this range we can hear, the easier it should be to learn to speak.*

The range of pitch and of loudness of all of our speech sounds together is called the "speech spectrum" **[pp. 78–89]**. The *speech spectrum,* when it is related to normal hearing, can be displayed on an audiogram form, as in Figure 5. If we recorded several people talking for several minutes, they would produce a wide range of pitch and loudness in their speech sounds. When this range is related to the way a normal ear hears different sounds, we can show on an audiogram form, like Figure 5, that the average level of the speech spectrum (shown by the dark line) is well beyond the normal hearing-threshold level (shown by the zero line on the audiogram), and would be easy to hear.

Some frequencies of speech are naturally farther beyond normal threshold (0 dB) than others. For example, the 500 Hertz part of speech averages 55 decibels greater than the hearing threshold while the 8000 Hertz part averages only 30 decibels more than normal hearing threshold. This difference in strength at different frequencies contributes to the "natural" sound of speech. If a hearing aid is to reproduce speech that sounds more natural, it is important that all of the frequencies of the speech spectrum are reproduced so that their natural differences in intensity are maintained. **[pp. 93–**

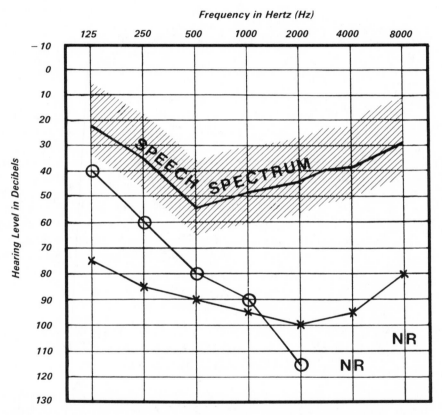

Figure 5. A pure-tone audiogram form showing the long-term average speech spectrum at a normal conversational level. Since the speech spectrum is at a level much greater than 0 dB (normal hearing-threshold level), the entire spectrum is heard by a normal ear. The hearing-threshold levels and audiometric configurations shown for the left ear (X) and right ear (O) of a person with severe-to-profound hearing level indicate that none of the unamplified speech spectrum is audible to either ear.

94] In other words, if we increased the sound of speech more noticeably above the hearing threshold at 8000 Hertz than at 500 Hertz, speech would sound very unnatural.

Before we go on examining the speech spectrum, notice that the threshold curves for either the right or left ear shown on Figure 5 are beyond the loudest part of the natural speech spectrum. A child who had hearing levels like this would not hear normal speech at all in either ear. Such a child might see the mouth moving but would not pick up any sound. If the speaker raised his voice, perhaps almost shouting, so that the entire speech spectrum was made louder, the child might hear the speech softly, but only in the right ear (marked with O), and would hear only the lower frequency components of speech so that it would sound distorted. *You might be able to arrange for an audiologist or teacher to let you hear such "filtered" speech so that you can see what happens to the speech spectrum when only part of it is audible.*

It is not good enough just to make the speech louder overall with a hearing aid because the speech would sound distorted to an impaired ear that doesn't hear some sounds as well as others. *The audiologist should try to see that the amplifier selected for each child reproduces the speech spectrum so that the child can hear as much of it as possible.* **[pp. 93–94]** In order to do this, a hearing aid will have to be selected that can be adjusted to make certain sounds louder than others. If possible, all the sounds of the speech spectrum should be amplified beyond the hearing-threshold level for the ear, but none should be beyond the tolerance level. Figure 6 shows a situation in which parts of the speech spectrum have been selectively amplified to hit the dynamic range target of a child's impaired left ear. Because the dynamic range is so narrow, the audiologist will need to be very skilled to do this for each ear.

IF SOUNDS CAN BE AMPLIFIED TO WITHIN THE DYNAMIC RANGE, WHY CAN'T MY CHILD UNDERSTAND SPEECH?

Even with the excellent fitting results shown in Figure 6, amplified speech will not sound natural. Notice that the average of the unamplified speech spectrum in the top portion of the audiogram form is well beyond normal hearing threshold—about 50 decibels greater than threshold through the "speech frequencies," and easy to hear. **[pp. 94–95]** But when the speech is amplified for the left ear in that example, the average can be only 10 or 15 decibels stronger than threshold. Otherwise speech sounds might exceed the tolerance level of that ear. *See if you can arrange for an audiologist or a school to let your hear speech that is presented to one of your ears at about 10 to 15 decibels above your threshold.* Would it

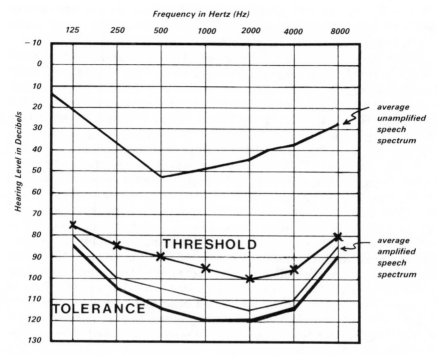

Figure 6. *Amplification of the average speech spectrum to reach the hearing level of the listener's left ear but not beyond the tolerance level. The amplified speech spectrum is reproduced relative to the listener's hearing level and tolerance level at each of the frequencies on the audiogram. Note that the listener's restricted dynamic range of hearing limits the intensity range around the average amplified speech spectrum.*

be difficult to attend and listen to speech at that soft level all day?

Notice, too, in Figure 6 that the narrow dynamic range in that example will not permit much *variation* in intensity around the average line of the speech spectrum. The original unamplified speech spectrum, displayed in Figure 5, has about a 30-decibel range from the softest to the loudest sounds at each of the frequencies. With speech amplified as illustrated in Figure 6, the range is squeezed into only approximately 20 decibels, and less at some frequencies. *Some normal variations in loudness will be missing and this will influence the understanding and naturalness of speech.*

Still another reason why children with severe hearing impairment cannot understand speech through their ear is *frequency distortion.* **[p. 93]** Look again at Figure 5 (page 23) and notice the *right* ear hearing-threshold levels indicated by the circles. While the threshold levels at 125 Hertz, 250 Hertz,

500 Hertz, and 1000 Hertz are actually better than for the left ear, the threshold at 2000 Hertz requires so much power that it may be very close to the child's tolerance level. Amplification of sounds of that frequency may not reach the right ear. When tested at 4000 Hertz and 8000 Hertz in this example, there was no response at all to these tones in the right ear. Sounds of those frequencies delivered to that ear, even at very strong levels, would not be heard. The right ear of this example will hear only the lower frequency sounds of speech through amplification. That is *frequency distortion.* While the right ear might receive parts of the amplified speech spectrum, it will not receive enough for a child to understand speech.

In addition, there is liable to be distortion in the child's impaired ear that will make sound unclear. **[pp. 73–75]** The child needs to be able to tell small differences in pitch and loudness in order to distinguish most speech sounds through listening. Experiments show that the greater the hearing impairment is the less able a person is to hear these important differences that contribute to the understanding of speech. We do not know for sure *what* a hearing-impaired child actually hears when we ask him to listen for a tone. For example, when the audiologist presented a 2000 Hertz tone to the right ear of the example in Figure 5, the child responded—but to what? Because of impairment in that ear causing sound distortion, the child might have heard a noise of many frequencies. *Just because a child responds to amplified tones of various frequencies does not always mean that the child actually heard those exact tones.*

WHAT GOOD IS A HEARING AID, IF THE LAST STATEMENT IS TRUE?

Plenty! Remember that we said that children do not need to hear all of the speech spectrum in order to use their hearing to help them *learn* and *monitor* their own speech. Children and adults do not need to hear all of the speech spectrum in order to use hearing to help *understand* speech, either. In everyday conversation, even with normal hearing, we seldom actually *hear* all of the speech sounds that are said because of noise in the background or distance from the speaker. There is a lot of information in speech that helps us *guess* what a sound might have been when we did not hear it for sure. For example, if you hear someone say "I'm going on a diet to get thinner," but you really didn't hear the first soft **th** sound in *thinner,* wouldn't you know that the sound must be **th**? That's part of what we learn about spoken language. It's called *redundancy* and we use it all the time to get along. The telephone companies know that, so to save money they do not transmit all of the speech signal over their wires. Try saying the words *fin* and *thin* over the telephone and see how well a listener can tell the difference. But if you mentioned one of those words in a sentence about *fish,* the listener would believe he actually heard the **f** sound in *fin.*

Hearing-impaired children also use the limited information they can get from amplified speech to accompany the limited information they can also get from watching the lips of the speaker. With a little information through the ear added to a little information through the eye, most hearing-impaired children can become very good lipreaders. Information through the ear + information through the eye = speechreading. Children also use facial expressions and observation of the situation to fill in some blanks in the speaker's message.

WHAT IS THE BEST TYPE OF AMPLIFIER FOR MY CHILD?

Although someone may tell you that this or that brand or a particular new kind of hearing aid or classroom amplifier is the best, none of the systems is superior in all situations. The following are the major kinds of amplification systems with some of their advantages and disadvantages! **[pp. 101–102]**

1. *The "hard-wire" group amplification system* is among the oldest in use in classrooms. It consists of one or more microphones wired to a large amplifying circuit that delivers sound by wires to several sets of earphones. It can have numerous controls and adjustments, and its primary advantages are its wide-frequency bandwith and powerful gain (sound amplification). But, it limits the child's mobility and is not available outside the classroom. Therefore, consistency of amplified sound is not possible. A smaller version of the hard-wire group system is the more portable "desk model." This can be moved from place to place, and can be adjusted to suit each student, but it is not a wearable device that can go everywhere and it usually has only one microphone for receiving speech.

2. *The wearable hearing aid* is probably the most common amplification system in use among hearing-impaired children, primarily because of its portability. It is available either as a bodyworn amplifier and microphone case with a cord leading to an earphone, or worn over and behind the ear. The wearable aid gives the greatest mobility and the possibility of a consistent amplified speech signal throughout the day. Since the microphone is on the child's own body, it can provide good feedback from his own speech. But its distance from other speakers admits unwanted noise, resulting in a poor speech signal-to-noise ratio. The separated microphones of two wearable aids also offer an opportunity for locating the source of sounds, especially when hearing aids are worn on the head to facilitate "searching" movements.

3. *Loop induction systems* use magnetic radiation from a microphone and transmitter, utilizing wires looped on the floor, often under a carpet. The child's wearable receiver picks up sound through magnetic radiation rather than from the air, amplifies it and sends it to the ear. When the microphone is close to the teacher's mouth, the child can receive the sound of her speech across the room without the interfering background noises of the classroom that would have been received through the air. The child's reception of sound amplified in this fashion is limited to classrooms equipped with loops of magnetic wire.

4. *Air broadcasting systems* provide the teacher with a microphone connected to a portable amplifier and transmitter, much like a miniature radio station. The child wears a receiver, like a small radio, tuned to the frequency of the teacher's transmitter. When the microphone is close to the teacher's mouth, the child can receive the sound across the room without the interference of background noise from the classroom that would have been received through a microphone located on the child. Such RF (Radio Frequency) or FM (Frequency Modulation) systems should include controls for using a microphone on the child's unit so that he can receive his own speech feedback.

Space-age technology suggests promising advances in providing amplification for deaf children by infra-red rays and perhaps laser beams. Repositioning of microphones and loud speakers, and increasingly compact circuitry hold promise for increasing "gain" without (sound amplification) feedback squeal in small hearing aids. The future looks very promising for improved systems of electro-acoustic amplification for hearing-impaired children.

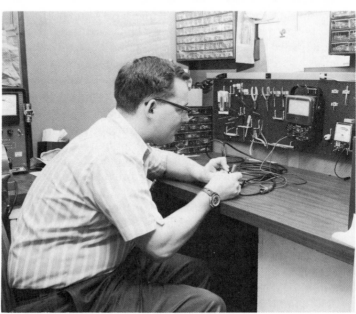

School technician checking a hearing aid.

CHAPTER IV

How Can You Help Your Child Use the Hearing He Still Possesses?*

Having your child's hearing carefully measured and selecting the best possible hearing aids are two important beginning steps—the subjects of the last two chapters. They are so important that you may not want to leave them just to chance, or completely in the hands of professionals. As parents, you can become careful and effective consumers of professional services and equipment. You should not let anyone tell you, "Your child is too young for a hearing test. Come back in six months and we'll see what we can do," or "He might use a hearing aid when he's older," or "There are schools for deaf children when they are old enough."

Here are some suggestions that may help you in dealing with these important beginning steps. WARNING: *they may make you unpopular with some of the professionals with whom you come in contact.* Remember, you will want to work cooperatively as part of a team with a number of different professionals—physicians, audiologists, speech pathologists, teachers—but *no one else* but you has the same special responsibility for your child.

---

*Bold face page references refer to: Calvert, Donald R. and Silverman, S. Richard, *Speech and Deafness,* Revised Edition, Washington, DC: Alexander Graham Bell Association for the Deaf, 1983.

HOW CAN YOU MAKE SURE THAT YOUR CHILD'S HEARING IS TESTED CORRECTLY?

First, you should make sure that the audiologist is competent. The American Speech-Language-Hearing Association (ASHA) grants *Certificates of Clinical Competence* (CCC) to audiologists, and such a certificate should be in evidence in the office or test room. The same association accredits clinics, centers, and programs that meet the basic requirements for giving audiology services, and you might want to ask to see the *accreditation* certificate.

Unfortunately, this doesn't guarantee that the person who is going to test your child's hearing is familiar with severely hearing-impaired or deaf children. Some audiologists go through their entire career without seeing a child or adult who has problems any more serious than being hard of hearing. You may have to ask about this! You may also wish to sit in and watch your child being tested if you can.

Next, you should see whether the clinic has suitable equipment for testing children with severe and profound hearing impairment. Remember, we said in Chapter 2 that not all audiometers were equipped for levels powerful enough to reach the hearing threshold of children with severe impairment. You may also ask about capability of testing for hearing up to 16000 Hertz to make sure your child isn't one of the few who has some "hidden" hearing in the very high frequencies. That requires special equipment. In addition, the hearing test equipment should be appropriate for the age of your child. Babies can be tested now from the first few days after birth with a threshold audiogram that is fairly accurate and helpful in selecting hearing aids. There are a number of devices that help an experienced audiologist get responses from infants, toddlers and very young children.

Once you have found a clinic or center where your child's hearing can be tested, and have found an audiologist in whom you have confidence, arrange to see that your child's hearing is tested at regular intervals. All hearing-impaired children should have a complete test at least once a year, and young children should be tested more often.

A few schools for hearing-impaired children have testing facilities and audiology services that are a built-in part of the school program. *More schools should have these!* There are published guidelines for audiology services in schools and classes for hearing-impaired children,* and you may want to ask your school staff if you can see them. The guidelines suggest one full-time audiologist for every 75 to 100 hearing-impaired children, and one hearing-aid technician for every 100 to 150 children. They also suggest the equipment that audiology programs should have.

---

*Ross, Mark and Calvert, Donald R., Guidelines for Audiology Programs in Educational Settings for Hearing-Impaired Children, *Volta Review,* 1977, *79,* 153–161.

WHAT ABOUT SELECTING HEARING AIDS?

In the last chapter we mentioned making sure there was enough *gain* so that speech was above your child's threshold but with a limiting control on the amount of power so that the hearing aid does not exceed your child's tolerance level with sudden loud noises. You might want to ask the audiologist to show you audiograms with this information for each of your child's ears. There are some other things to watch for, too. *You should make sure that your child can hear his own speech through the hearing aid,* since that will help him monitor the speech he produces. **[pp. 96–97]** One amplifier may be better than another for this purpose. Ask your audiologist to test for this.

No matter how well an amplifier improves the sound, it won't be of much benefit unless it is comfortable for your child to wear. **[pp. 99–100]** Some big wearable units weigh too much for a two or three-year-old to wear throughout the day. Amplifying units with tight earphones worn on the head can be very uncomfortable on a child's outer ear, and do no better job than some softer insert earmolds. Some of the old superstitions, for example, "in order for a medicine to be *good*, it must taste *bad*," may still be applied to hearing devices, but neither the largest nor the most expensive instrument is necessarily the best.

A hearing aid, particularly for active young children, should permit a child to move about without being hindered in most of his daily activities. It is difficult to learn language or any other subject if you are confined to the desk or table where your amplifier is located. If a child has to take off his hearing aid every time he leaves a room, his teacher is likely to see that he doesn't have to leave the room very often.

A hearing aid should be simple to operate. **[p. 100]** If *you* can't manage it, you should not expect *your child* to do so. And you should work toward having your child take care of his own hearing aid. Make sure the controls are large enough and easy to understand, and that the battery can be changed by little hands. If not, complain to the companies that manufacture these aids.

HOW DO YOU MAKE SURE YOUR CHILD USES HIS HEARING ALL THE TIME?

Just because children wear heaing aids doesn't mean they are necessarily using their hearing. **[pp. 102–105]** Remember the old saying, "You can't judge a book by its cover." In some recent experiments when audiologists made sudden inspections of hearing-impaired children in classrooms, a large number of the children were getting very little or nothing from their hearing aids. *What went wrong?* Some of the children weren't even wearing their hearing aids because they were in the shop for repair and wouldn't be back for several weeks. Others simply had forgotten to wear them. When the hearing aids that were being worn were examined, some of them did not have batteries in them or the batteries were very weak, cords were broken, parts were broken or missing, or the aids were distorting sound very badly. Sometimes the ear mold didn't fit or the gain dial had not been set properly. Then too, some of the children had wax in their ear canals so that the amplified sound could not reach the ear. **[p. 45]** A few children had middle-ear infections so that the additional hearing loss made their hearing aid ineffective.

Something certainly had gone wrong! It made no difference how well hearing had been measured, how carefully the hearing aid had been selected, or how much parents paid for the hearing aids. It made no difference, either, how skillful parents or classroom teachers might be in stimulating the children's hearing. Something was missing!

What was missing was a *system* or program that assures that children always get the maximum benefit from their hearing aids **[pp. 102–105]** That doesn't happen naturally! It won't be easy! The combined efforts of home, clinic, and school are needed to make it work. *But the basic principle underlying the use of hearing for developing, improving, and maintaining speech is that amplified speech must be constantly available so that the child can rely on its use.* To assure constancy of amplified speech, a program of careful monitoring is needed—one that goes well beyond just seeing that the child "has on his hearing aid" every morning.

Here are some essentials of a beneficial monitoring program:

1. *Regular Hearing Evaluation*

A complete hearing evaluation of each child should be performed by an audiologist at the beginning of each school year. Middle-ear impedance tests should be conducted at this time, as well as those measures that describe the child's hearing capabilities and assist in hearing aid selection and fitting. Evaluation of the child's use of amplification should also be made, especially for feedback of the child's own speech. In order to establish this *beginning-of-the-year hearing baseline* for a large group of children within the first few weeks of school, it may be necessary to begin audiologic evaluations for some children during the summer, before the starting day of school. A hearing-screening evaluation should be performed after the children return from their midwinter recess. In cold climates where ear infections may be more prevalent, this *midyear evaluation* and other evaluations during the year should be compared with those of the baseline evaluation.

2. *Regular Hearing Aid Evaluation*

An electro-acoustic examination of each hearing aid should be conducted *at the beginning of each school year,* and then no less than once a month throughout the school year. Records of the gain, maximum power output, frequency response, and distortion characteristics should be kept for each hearing aid or classroom amplifier, and placed in a card file or computer so that changes in the response of each hearing aid can be observed. Significant changes in an amplifier are indications for preventive maintenance or replacement.

Each morning, a parent, teacher, dormitory counselor, or some other person appointed for this purpose should check the hearing aid by a listening test through an ear insert or other device, then check the level of the battery, and also check the cord connections for intermittency. This daily test should be carried out as carefully on *weekends* as on school days. During summer vacation periods, the parents should maintain the regular morning tests of hearing aids, and arrange repair as needed with the school, clinic or hearing aid distributor. The teacher who first works with the child each day, and the parents on weekends, should also observe the child's responses to amplification by using some simple behavioral tests. Your teacher or audiologist can suggest some for you to use. As early as possible, all children should be taught to conduct their own tests of their hearing aid batteries, and to listen carefully in order to judge whether the hearing aid is working satisfactorily.

3. *Regular Examination of Outer Ear, Ear Canal and Earmold*

At least weekly, a special effort should be made by the parents, school nurse, audiologist, or other person appointed for this purpose, to examine each child's ear canals for obvious accumulation of wax and for irritation, and the outer ear for signs of irritation from the earmold. Each earmold should be cleaned and examined at that time, including a check of its seal with the receiver or tubing. Abnormal feedback squeal should be reported and the cause determined. New earmolds should be made as needed.

4. *Emergency Hearing and Amplification Services*

Those times when a child is either without regular amplification or when the child is not responding well to sound should be treated as *educational emergencies,* whenever teaching speech depends upon using hearing. Accordingly, a number of emergency services should be readily available near the location where children are taught, *preferably on the school campus.* These should include immediate electro-acoustic examinations of the amplifier or hearing aid when it is not functioning well or when the child is not responding to amplified sound in his customary manner. If the amplifier is not working properly, the parents or school should arrange to have the aid repaired by a technician *on the premises,* or should arrange to have available a similar instrument that can be borrowed while the child's own aid is being repaired. A reasonable target is for children not to be deprived of their customary amplification *longer than one hour* during any day. During the summer and vacation periods, parents will need to arrange these same emergency services.

When it is discovered that a child is not responding to sound as well as he usually does but the hearing aid is in good operating condition, an immediate hearing evaluation should be conducted. This should include tests for middle-ear function and inspection of the ear canal, considering the possibility of infection or of something impeding the transmission of sound through the middle ear. Medical referral should be made as needed.

5. *Efficient Medical Referral Services*

Middle-ear infections seem to be frequent among hearing-impaired children, particularly children under the age of 8 years. Closure of the ear canal by earmolds or muffs reduces ventilation to the skin of the ear. With chronic ear infections or draining ears, the actual time a child uses amplification may be severely reduced. A slight reduction in hearing, caused by temporary middle-ear impairment, may push the child's hearing threshold beyond the regularly set gain of his hearing aid. Arrangements should be made in advance with the family and the child's physicians, or with a school physician, to have an efficient medical referral system so that a hearing-impaired child wearing amplification can receive *priority treatment.* The importance of avoiding extended periods when the child is not receiving appropriate amplified speech will need to be made clear.

All this monitoring of hearing should be made part of your child's Individual Educational Program (IEP) provided by the school. You may have to urge your school to see that the program is carried out. However, the school cannot take responsibility for the many hours a child is not in the classroom. You know that most of any child's day will be spent outside the classroom. And even children who stay in school dormitories will spend many important days at home. *Your child's "hearing year" and "learning year" are 365 days long.* Here is a fine opportunity for parents to work closely with teachers and other school staff to see that an effective hearing-monitoring program is maintained. You and the school might even want to arrange some spontaneous sudden "spot checks," like fire drills, to see how well the auditory monitoring system is working at home and in the classroom.

You can easily see that there is a lot that you, as parents, can do. But one of the most important things you can do for your hearing-impaired child is to select a good school where teaching speech is not only a commitment, but where the staff knows how to teach it. The next chapter may help you do this.

CHAPTER V

What Happens When They Teach Speech in School?*

In the first chapter of this book we gave some reasons why hearing-impaired children don't talk naturally, why they have to be *taught* to speak, instead. A few especially talented parents have undertaken to teach their own children, following advice from others and using their own common sense. Some have taken special training and become teachers, themselves. But most parents look to schools or clinics for instructors who have made a profession of teaching hearing-impaired children.

Pioneering teachers improved their skill by experience, getting better throughout their careers with each new child they taught, and developing techniques by trial and error. The teachers that followed learned their craft largely by watching master teachers—by learning "on the job" as apprentices until they, too, became master teachers. Special teacher-training programs became more common after World War II. It has been only in recent years that the knowledge gained by skilled teachers has been systematically written down in such books as *Speech and Deafness* so that important ideas can be relayed to future generations, and it is only recently also that most teachers of hearing-impaired children have been prepared through college courses combined with supervised practice teaching.

---

*Bold face references in text refer to: Calvert, Donald R. and Silverman, S. Richard, *Speech and Deafness*, Revised Edition, Washington, DC: Alexander Graham Bell Association for the Deaf, 1983.

Meanwhile, scientific and technological progress has made some of the older "tried and true" methods obsolete. This is happening in almost every profession, industry, and trade. *The rate of progress is so fast now that today's student teachers will probably have to change the way they go about teaching speech several times during a career.* Advances in medical care seem to be changing the causes of deafness among children in our schools and that could influence the kind of problems they have with learning. **[p. 44]** Hearing aids and amplifiers are among the major technological advances that change teaching, and more improvements are on the way. Wearable devices that convert speech sounds to vibrations on the skin of even the very deafest children look promising in the near future. **[pp. 24–25]** Computers may change the way we provide practice on skills and introduce new information to children.

With these changes it probably will be harder for parents to judge whether they have found a good teacher or good school program for their child.

HOW CAN YOU TELL A GOOD TEACHER OR A GOOD PROGRAM WHEN YOU SEE ONE?

Parents will have to use careful observation and some uncommonly good common sense in judging how effective a teacher is. Certification of professional training programs and of teachers by such national organizations as the Council on Education of the Deaf (CED)* insure minimum standards for teachers, but they can't really guarantee skill or that a teacher has kept up with the times. *Teachers of speech are people. They seem to be "born" as well as "made."* That is, some teachers seem to have a natural ability to work with children and if given appropriate training can apply that ability to teaching speech right away. Others have a difficult time at first but then "blossom" with experience to become good, solid teachers. Still others seem never to be very good at it, however good their training might have been or how much experience they may have had. A teacher who has taught twenty years may have had one year of experience repeated twenty times. A few teachers seem to be able to work very well independently, without a supervised program and without other teachers or clinicians around, but most teachers work best where they are part of an organized program. Some teachers will be able to work very competently with their children but not "come across well" when they try to explain or demonstrate to parents or other adults what they are doing. And some will be able to verbalize what

---

*Write for information to the Council on Education of the Deaf (CED), Committee on Professional Preparation and Certification, c/o The Alexander Graham Bell Association for the Deaf, Information Services, 3417 Volta Place, N.W., Washington, D.C. 20007, telephone: (202) 337-5220, Voice or TTY.

they are doing, or should be doing, very well, but may not be able to carry it out with a class of children.

Visit classes and observe, if you can, in order to judge the quality of a school or other educational program. Most schools, classes and clinics will welcome your sitting in to see their work at first hand. Plan to spend at least one full day during regular school sessions in order to get a good sample, and see the children outside of class or wherever else they spend their school day. Be ready with some questions and take notes so that you can compare the programs you visit. Hearing-impaired children are taught speech in a variety of settings—in special schools where teaching speech is blended in with the teaching of classroom subjects; in regular or special classes, where speech teachers take them out of the classroom for a special "speech period" individually or in a small group; or in clinics where they work with a tutor "one-on-one" for several periods a week while they attend school elsewhere. You may find the variety of possibilities for educational placement of your hearing-impaired child sometimes confusing, but that variety can be useful in handling the variety of special abilities or difficulties hearing-impaired children seem to have.

Whatever the educational setting, there are some things that any good program should include for helping your child learn speech. In Chapter 4 we mentioned some requirements for getting the most out of whatever still exists of a child's hearing, and you may want to ask about the auditory monitoring program the school regularly provides to assure that the children's hearing aids are working at full capacity. When you are observing, see if all the children have amplification and use their hearing aids outside the classroom. Visit the school's audiologist and hearing-aid technician.

If children are taught in classes, check on size of the class and note the teacher/pupil ratio. Also, check to see whether instruction is individualized. **[pp. 54–55]** In other words, see if children in classes are grouped according to their speech ability during special speech periods, or whether they remain in the same class for speech, language, and all other school subjects. See whether teachers know the differences in individual children's hearing ability. If they have a special speech teacher, see how that work is tied in to what is happening in the classroom. For every six to ten teachers in a special school, there should be a supervising or coordinating teacher who sees that there is consistency and continuity of instruction for a group of children, and that teachers have help and advice when they need it. **[p. 64]** The school principal should manage the transfer of children from department to department.

One important thing you should consider doing for the benefit of your hearing-impaired child is to have an *Independent Educational Evaluation* (IEE) completed about every two years to measure overall progress in school. Speech development should be part of this IEE, as well as language development and academic progress. These comprehensive evaluations can be arranged at a few clinics and schools in various parts of the country, and should be scheduled in a different clinic or school than the one your child attends.* The "All Handicapped Children Act of 1975," Public Law 94-142, recommends this Independent Educational Evaluation, although it is not as well known as other parts of that landmark legislation.

WHAT ARE THE DIFFERENCES IN APPROACHES TO TEACHING SPEECH?

You may encounter different methods or systems of teaching that feature one or another distinctive techniques. Be wary of programs that depend too heavily upon a special electronic device, visual display gadget, or mysterious and complex piece of equipment that seems to work miracles *without the aid of good teaching.* [pp. 58-63] Such devices have come and gone with regularity in the history of educating hearing-impaired children. Ask about a program's philosophy of communication and approach to teaching speech. Don't be satisfied with such responses as "we use the (name of a person) method." Ask what that means!

Here are three major approaches commonly used in teaching hearing-impaired children to talk that may help you understand the many apparently conflicting methods and systems that you may see or about which you may hear. [pp. 115-152] A large school or program may beneficially utilize all three of these approaches, or select parts of the approaches to suit the different needs and capabilities of the range of children they teach. They may be able to shift appropriately from one to the other as a child progresses, either to help a child who runs into special problems, or to speed a child along who is learning very well.

1. *The primarily auditory approach*

Schools, classes and clinics that use this approach rely very heavily upon amplification of speech by individual hearing aids or classroom amplifiers to provide hearing-impaired children with speech stimulation that will encourage them to acquire speech. [pp. 116-130] Teaching procedures emphasize children learning how to listen and imitate what they hear, and then trying their own production of connected spoken language, rather than teaching each of the speech sounds directly. Some programs using this approach insist that the child be enrolled in a regular class with normal-hearing children, while auditory training and speech work is carried out in a clinic outside of school with a special tutor for each child. Hearing aids are worn constantly with an auditory monitoring

---

*Geers, Ann E., Moog, Jean S. and Calvert, Donald R., The Independent Educational Evaluation, *Volta Review,* 1980, *82,* 280–287.

program that includes the parents. Starting such a program very early, usually before the child is 3 years old, is thought to be essential. Phrases and sentences are the usual units of spoken language, although some practice is with syllables. **[p. 134]**

2. *The multi-sensory approach*

Those who use this approach believe that the impaired ear, even with the most modern amplification and the best auditory monitoring program, is not a sufficient avenue for teaching speech to most hearing-impaired children. **[pp. 130–145]** Those with a narrow dynamic range, as shown in the example of Figure 6 of Chapter 3 (page 25), for example, will receive limited speech information through the ear and can benefit from additional speech information conveyed through other sensory avenues—mainly what they can *see* and what they can *feel.* Speech needs to be taught more directly. Good programs that use this approach, usually in special schools, insist on amplification and auditory monitoring programs, but also teach speech by showing children how sounds are formed and letting them feel vibration on the skin or the flow of air as sounds are produced. The sculpture on the cover of this book represents an adult using vibration on the skin to stimulate the child to imitate production of voice. Effective teachers are selective in the sensory avenues they use to teach various units of speech—sometimes emphasizing hearing, sometimes vision, sometimes touch, or a combination of all three. **[pp. 58–60]** The teacher works directly with each child on speech sounds for practice in syllables, words and sentences. Speech training and usage is woven into other subjects taught in school throughout the day, and the school depends heavily upon parents for carry-over of speech in real communication situations at home.

3. *The sound-by-sound association approach*

This is usually reserved for hearing-impaired children who have additional learning problems or who have not been successful in learning by either of the first two approaches. **[pp. 145–149]** It takes advantage of whatever sensory avenue is needed to teach a child to *produce* carefully and individually each of the speech sounds. Then the child is taught to *write* the common alphabet symbol for that sound, to *recognize the symbol by sight* and say the associated sound, to *lipread* the speech sound as it is produced by the teacher and other children, and to *recognize the sound by listening,* providing the child's hearing is good enough. Each of the consonant and vowel sounds are taught in this manner and are nearly mastered before new sounds are learned. When the child is able to say, write, read, lipread and listen for most of the speech sounds, they are combined into syllables and words, and associated with meaning. Words, in turn, are said, written, read, lipread and recognized through hearing before they are grouped into sentences which are associated with mean-

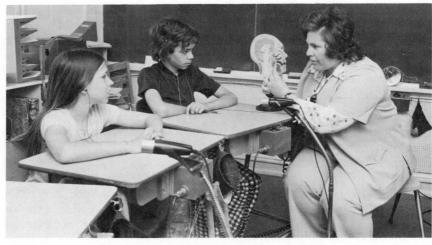

Explaining speech structures and terms.

ing. Some hearing-impaired children seem to need this slower, more analytic approach, that emphasizes associated written symbols very early.

WHAT DOES A TEACHER OF HEARING-IMPAIRED CHILDREN NEED TO KNOW?

In preparation for teaching speech, the teacher needs a combination of: (1) basic knowledge, (2) techniques for teaching, and (3) supervised practice with children. The areas of basic knowledge or foundation courses should include *anatomy* and physiology of human speech and hearing mechanisms, *audiology* and amplification of sound, *phonetics* and analysis of speech, and *psychology* that has to do with the principles of learning speech and language. Here is a brief review of each of these.

Anatomy

The teacher of speech is particularly interested in the parts of the body where speech sounds are produced. **[pp. 16–20]** The structures of the mouth and throat, and how these parts function to make the sounds that transmit our spoken language, should be familiar to teachers. Figure 7 shows some of the more important parts of the speech mechanism. Teachers may need, for example, to show a child how a speech sound like the t in *too* is produced. **[pp. 184–185]** They will know that the front part of the tongue presses close against the alveolar ridge (the gum ridge just behind the upper front teeth) and is then released with a brief explosion of air from the lungs. Competent speech teachers will need to be so familiar with anatomy associated with speech production that they can listen to a child's speech, tell how and why an incorrect unit of speech was produced, produce the unit themselves, and show the child how the speech unit should be produced. **[p. 241]**

Audiology

Chapters 2, 3, and 4 of this book outlined some basic things teachers will need to know about audiology and amplification of sound. **[pp. 68–105]** Of course, they should have the audiograms of each child *readily available* and know how they relate to understanding and producing speech. Teachers should be familiar with the terms and tests that audiologists are likely to use with the hearing-impaired children they teach, and should be able to explain these terms and tests to you. They will also need to know about classroom acoustics—how to reduce and control noise that might otherwise get into a child's hearing aid and interfere with the proper hearing of speech. **[pp. 45–99]**

Phonetics

The speech teacher will be specifically concerned with the children's voices, their use of speech rhythm, and their articulation. **[pp. 20–39]** The

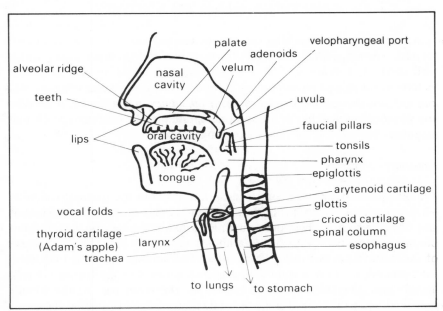

Figure 7. Diagram of structures used in speech production.

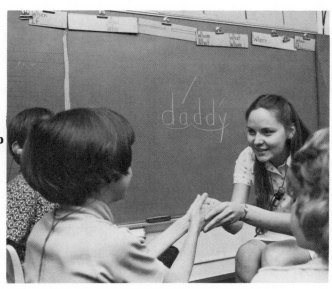

Clapping the hands to develop appreciation for accent.

voice should be loud enough to carry the speech message to listeners, and be set at a comfortable pitch level that is easy to listen to. Resonance of the voice should not be overly nasal, with the back of the throat open to the nasal cavity, except for the **m, n** and **ng** sounds. **[pp. 216–221]** *Rhythm* of phrases and sentences should be similar to that of children with normal hearing. "Accent," for example, is the stress we place on a syllable within a word. Try pronouncing these common words with the wrong accent as indicated: *América, sylláble, ábove, intéresting*. Notice how hard they are to understand that way.

It is useful to have written symbols to point to when we are talking to children about the various speech sounds of *articulation*. **[pp. 8–16]** It is best if these symbols are from our own alphabet, and even better if they could help children "sound out" words for reading. Unfortunately, our alphabet has only 26 letters to represent the 43 different speech sounds we commonly produce when we speak. The sound of **f**, for example, may be spelled "f" (*fir*), "ff" (*differ*), "ph" (*phone*), "gh" (*rough*) or "lf" (*half*). Think how the letter "o" changes in these words: *ton, top, told, tomb, woman, women*.

"Phoneticians," those who study speech, use a system of written symbols that include some Greek and Old English letters, called the *I*nternational *P*honetic *A*lphabet (IPA). **[p. 9]** Dictionaries give us markings to indicate the pronunciation of words. Teachers commonly use a simplified system of alphabet symbols to indicate to children what speech sounds they are talking about in practice or when correcting attempts at speech. One system is called the General American Speech and Phonic Symbols. They are shown with key words in Table 3. **[pp. 12–16]**

Symbol	***Pronounced as in***	***Symbol***	***Pronounced as in***
p	pie	$\overset{1}{th}$	thin
b	by	$\overset{2}{th}$	then
t	tie	zh	vision
d	day	qu	queen
k	key	x	box
g	go		
h	he	ee	bee
wh	why	-i-	bit
f	fan	-e-	bet
v	vine	-a-	bat
s	see	oo	too
z	zoo	-oo-	foot
sh	she	aw	lawn
ch	chin	-o-	top
j	jam	-u-	cup
m	me	ur	burn
n	no	oi	coin
ng	long	ou	mouth
y-	yes	oa	boat
l	lie	u-e	cute
r	red	a-e	made
w-	we	i-e	time

Table 3. Speech symbols with key words for pronunciation.

Children learn that when the teacher writes these symbols, they always mean the same speech sounds. The dashes show the position of some sounds in a word. For example, the *-i-* is between the letters "b" and "t" in *bit*. The small numeral ^{1} just above the *th* means that the sound is made without voice (as in *thin*), and the numeral ^{2} means that the sound is made with voice (as in *then*). The ^{1} always means the sound is voiceless. The ^{2} always means the sound is voiced.

Sometimes knowing these symbols helps children "sound out" a new word. For example, a child may be able to pronounce the word *trade,* even though it is not familiar, by observing that it is made up of a sequence of the *t r a-e d* sounds. Not all of our words are so predictable, though, and teachers or parents may need to use the symbols to show how an unusual new word should be said. A child may be able to say *psychology,* for example, if we write the speech symbols just above the letters and cross out the silent letter "p."

si-ekolujee
p̸sychology

The numerals are useful for showing whether a sound is voiced or not by writing one of them above the letter, as in *cats*[1] and *dogs*[2].

To help with reading, older children learn several other rules. For example, they learn that the letter "c" followed by "a" or "o" or "u" is usually pronounced **k** as in *cat, cot* and *cut,* but when "c" is followed by "i" or "e" or "y" it is commonly pronounced **s** as in *city, cent* and *cycle.* They also learn that "ph" is commonly said **f** as in *phone,* that the letter "n" followed by "k" is pronounced **ng** as in *ink,* and that the final letter "y" is usually said **ee** as in *busy.*

Teachers learn not only *about* these speech sounds but learn ways to teach them. As an example of the information and procedures a teacher might have available, see the reprinted section of *Speech and Deafness* that deals with the sound of **k**. Note the information about this sound's production, feedback information, and other sensory information that might be useful for teaching; **[pp. 187–190]** the suggestions for development that follow an order from natural-to-more-complex techniques; **[p. 55]** the common errors for that sound, and suggestions for correcting or improving the sound when errors occur. The **k** sound is particularly difficult for hearing-impaired children to produce.

KEY WORDS: key, ba**c**k, be**c**ome
SPELLINGS: k, c, -ck, cc,
ch(school), -(a)lk

k   /k/   k

Production (*lingua-velar voiceless stop*)

STOP: No voice, velopharyngeal port closes, back of tongue closes against front portion of velum or back portion of palate, air is held and compressed in the back of the oral cavity. *Note:* the point of contact on the velum-palate changes with surrounding vowels.

EXPLOSION: Air compressed in the back of the oral cavity is exploded as audible breath between the velum-palate and back of the tongue through slightly open teeth and lips.

In connected speech, **k** is stopped but not exploded preceding **s** (*cooks, talks*) or another stop consonant in the same syllable (*act, elect*), and following **s** in the same syllable (*skin, scat*). It is exploded in the initial position of words and syllables (*king, crow, declare*), and immediately following any consonant in the final position (*ask, bank, bark, milk*). It is either not exploded or very lightly exploded in the final position following a vowel (*like, sack*).

Internal Feedback Information

TACTILE: Closure of back of tongue on velum or palate gives little information.

KINESTHETIC: Raising of back of tongue to close against velum or palate gives little information.

Sensory Instructional Possibilities

TACTILE: Exploded air on skin of the hand.

VISUAL: Exploded air by movement of feather, flame, or paper; place of production visible only with exaggerated mouth opening.

Suggestions for Development

1. Imitate from teacher's model; *avoid* dropping jaw with production. *Note:* fair to very poor sensory features make **k** a difficult sound to develop from imitation.

2. Demonstrate manner of production by analogy from **p** and **t**.

3. Demonstrate explosion by tactile impression of breath on student's hand.

4. Demonstrate explosion by visual impression of sudden movement of strip of paper, feather, or candle flame; *avoid* exaggeration of force of articulation.

5. Demonstrate place of production by slowly giving a visual exaggeration of the formation: with the teacher's mouth wide open, place the back of the tongue against the back portion of the palate (keeping the tip of the tongue behind the lower front teeth), slowly narrow mouth opening (keeping tongue in place) toward normal position and explode **k**. Have student attempt to imitate this production, using a mirror if necessary.

6. Demonstrate manner and place of production by giving a visually exaggerated step-by-step production: form **k** with the back of the tongue against the back of the upper front teeth (keeping the tip of the tongue behind the lower front teeth and explode (sound will be similar to **t**); next make the closure with the back of the tongue on the alveolar ridge and explode; next closure on the front portion of the palate and finally on the back portion of the palate. Have the student imitate each step as the back of the tongue is drawn back into the oral cavity.

7. Develop **k** in association with the **ee** vowel, a position in which the tongue is very close to the velum-palate, helping to avoid dropping the jaw on production of **k**. Closure of the **k** on syllables **eek** or **kee** is likely to be at the back of the palate rather than on the velum, avoiding unwanted noise of closure on the back of the velum and uvula.

8. While the student attempts to produce **t**, hold the tip of his tongue down (with finger or tongue blade) behind the lower front teeth (do not let the back of the tongue move forward). Associate the exploded sound he produces with written "k." After several repetitions with the teacher or student holding down the tip of the tongue, have the student attempt the production without this aid.

9. Have the seated student hold his mouth slightly open and breathe deeply through his nose (to accomplish this the velum and back of tongue must make closure). See that the tip of the tongue lies against the lower front teeth. While expelling breath through his nose, have student occlude his nostrils quickly with his thumb and forefinger, forcing the air to separate the velum and back of the tongue. Associate with written "k"; repeat.

10. Have the student lie on his back, relaxed (in this position the velum and back of the tongue are very close together). Have student breathe through his slightly opened mouth and attempt **k** explosion. *Note:* production will occur far back on the velum and should later be brought forward.

11. Develop the unreleased **k** after the exploded production is accomplished. Demonstrate with techniques similar to those suggested for the sound **p.**

12. If necessary, place teacher's thumb and forefinger on student's throat just under back of the tongue; press upward and forward, then move down quickly. Demonstrate explosion on teacher's production and ask student to attempt the same using his own thumb and forefinger on his throat.

Common Errors and Suggestions for Improvement

1. Excess or insufficient pressure on explosion of breath: Demonstrate as with **p** and **t**. Reduce pressure by having student produce a series of rapid **k** sounds (**kkkkkkkkkk**) on one breath, then produce syllables **kee kee kee kee kee** on another single breath.

2. Lack of closure for stop: Demonstrate by analogy with **p** and **t**. Have student produce series of **ptk** (**ptkptkptkptkptk**) on a single breath. Demonstrate difference between steady breath and sudden explosion with strip of paper or other visual aid. Redevelop in syllables following **ng**: extend **ng** and stop with breath (whispered) explosion. Use visual aids as needed. If **k** closure is accomplished in syllables, tell student to make n̍g without voice and then produce **k** at the end of the syllable.

3. Closure made too far back on velum and tongue: With diagrams compare correct and incorrect placement. Have student keep tip of tongue against lower front teeth while producing **k**. Practice **k** in syllables with **ee** and other vowels with forward tongue placement.

*4. Substitution of **g** for **k**, a sonant for surd error:* Write "g" and cross out to make student aware of nature of error. Demonstrate tactile difference as with **b** for **p**, and **d** for **t**. Extend duration of exploded **k** as with **p** and **t**.

5. Mouth too far open: Redevelop, demonstrating that the jaw does not drop on production. Use mirror or, if necessary, place hand under student's jaw on production of a series of **kkkkkkkkkk**. Develop in association with vowel **ee**; use exercises such as **eekee, eekee, eekee,** using a mirror to show that the mouth opening is very slight. Place a pencil or tongue blade between the teeth and have student produce **k**, without letting go of object.

6. Explosion made as glottal stop: Redevelop by analogy from **p** and **t**, moving back from **p** to **t** to **k**, and showing place of production by exaggerating if necessary.

Psychology

People who scientifically observe how we learn speech, in the expanding field of "psycho-linguistics," recognize different phases as a child with normal hearing is learning to talk. These phases, presented in Table 4, are useful for teachers in planning the sequence of activities for teaching hearing-impaired children to speak. **[pp. 107–110]** Observers of speech development also note that children with normal hearing do not acquire all of the speech sounds at the same time. Some seem to be learned very early and others come much later. In Figure 8, you can see that the **f** sound typically begins to be controlled at age two and is mastered by most children by age four, while the similar **v** sound begins later at age four and isn't under good control for most children until age eight. This suggests that the teacher should attempt to teach hearing-impaired children the **f** sound before the **v** sound, and not try to have the child master the **v** sound very early.

Motivation is essential for learning anything, including speech. The teacher should motivate speech, not as an end in itself, but as a skill needed for social experience and self enrichment. **[pp. 47–50]** The following are general rules, from a well known psychologist, that teachers keep in mind about motivation:

1. *A motivated learner acquires what he learns more readily than one who is not motivated. Motives include both general and specific ones—*

Phase 1. Input of sounds and spoken language are directed to the child by adults without observable responses, particularly vocal responses, being expected of the child.

Phase 2. The child begins to imitate the spoken language of the adults who talk to him, repeating as best he can the sequence of speech sounds and speech rhythm he hears.

Phase 3. The child responds to the spoken language of the adults who talk to him, not merely imitating what they say, but by answering with a different vocal response.

Phase 4. The child initiates speech sounds or spoken language without the immediate, associated stimulus of an adult speech model, talking to himself or initiating conversation with the adult.

Table 4. Four phases in learning spoken language for children with normal hearing in a sequence relevant for teaching speech to hearing-impaired children.

for example, desire to learn, need for achievement (general), desire for a reward, or desire to avoid a threatened punishment (specific).

2. *Learning through intrinsic (self) motivation is preferable to learning under extrinsic motivation.*

3. *Tolerance for failure is best taught through providing a backlog of success that compensates for the failure experienced.*

4. *Individuals need practice in setting realistic goals for themselves, goals neither so low as to require little effort nor so high as to encourage failure.*

5. *The personal history of the individual may hamper or enhance his ability to learn from a given teacher; for example, his reaction to authority.*

6. *Active participation by a student is preferable to passive reception when learning, for example, from a lecture or a motion picture.*

7. *Meaningful materials and meaningful tasks are learned more readily than nonsense materials and more readily than tasks not understood by the student.*

8. *There is no substitute for repetitive practice in the "over-learning" of skills.*

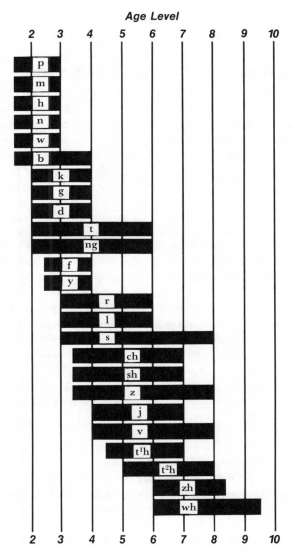

Figure 8. *Age levels at which children with normal hearing usually master the production of consonant sounds (see Table 3, p. 43 for speech symbols with key words for pronunciation). Adapted from Sander, E., When are speech sounds learned?,* Journal of Speech and Hearing Disorders, *1972, 37, 55–63.*

9. *Information about the nature of good performance, knowledge of one's own mistakes, and knowledge of successful results aid learning.*

10. *Reviews and reminders at regular intervals are helpful in fixing material that should be retained for a long time.*

WHAT SPECIAL EQUIPMENT FOR THE HEARING IMPAIRED DO THEY USE IN SCHOOLS?

We've already talked about the most important equipment—the hearing aid or classroom amplifier. There are some other sensory aids in use. We have mentioned devices that convert sound waves into vibration on the skin. These tactile aids are especially useful for children whose hearing impairment is very severe. Of course the skin is not nearly as good as the ear in discriminating subtle differences of frequency and intensity, but tactile information can particularly help a child monitor his voice. Engineering developments are continuing toward producing a wearable tactile device that deaf children can keep with them throughout the day.

There have been many sensory aids developed for hearing-impaired children that convert sound into something visible. **[pp. 62–63]** Sometimes it is the movement of the needle on a gauge, or lights that come on or move in response to different frequencies or intensities. The simplest device is a light bulb wired to a microphone and amplifier—when speech or other noise is present, the bulb goes on. This may be useful in getting a child to start vocalizing, or to help an older child adjust the loudness of his voice as he talks to a person at some distance.

Some of the visual sensory aids are very complex and very expensive. They all usually have the disadvantage of not being wearable so that a child can't use them outside of the clinic or classroom. Their success has generally been temporary.

The major sensory aid for teaching speech, in addition to the hearing aid, is the *teacher's or the parent's face.* It provides a combined sound and visible movement of the lips. **[pp. 59–60]** In addition, the child can feel the vibration on the face with his fingers, and pick up the flow of air from the speaker's mouth. It doesn't cost anything to buy, doesn't wear out, and seldom needs major repair. But its special merit is that it can give the child a most important reward—a smile of approval.

In this chapter, and in previous ones, I have purposely set some very high standards for school and clinic programs to follow. It is quite possible that you will hear "that's unrealistic" or "that would cost too much for us to do" or "no one has time for all that." When you hear that the expenditure of money or time is "not worth the effort," remember how a *self-fulfilling prophecy* works (see Chapter 2). Remember also that *parents* were responsible for starting the first schools for hearing-impaired children, and that *parents* have often led the drive for reform and improvement in schools. A great share of the responsibility for your hearing-impaired child's education rests with you, as described in the next chapter.

CHAPTER VI

What Can *You* Do To Help Your Child Use and Improve His Speech?*

If you have read this far, you have already done a lot. That's because understanding speech and deafness, and how speech is taught, is an important step. You may want to go further by reading some of the pages of *Speech and Deafness* suggested in the bracketed page numbers throughout this book.* Your school staff, speech pathologist, or audiologist may suggest some additional reading, and the Alexander Graham Bell Association for the Deaf in Washington, D.C., maintains a list of publications that are especially interesting to parents. See *Suggested Readings*, p. 61.

HOW CAN WE REALLY UNDERSTAND ABOUT SPEECH AND DEAFNESS?

There are things that parents might benefit from *knowing first-hand,* not just knowing them from what you have read or what you have been told. These suggestions to familiarize you with hearing and with speech may bring you closer to understanding what your child is experiencing. You will

*Bracketed page numbers in the text refer to: Calvert, Donald R. and Silverman, S. Richard, *Speech and Deafness,* Revised Edition, Washington, DC: Alexander Graham Bell Association for the Deaf, 1983 for additional reading on these topics.

need to have the help of your school or your hearing clinic, or ask your teacher or audiologist how these exercises might be arranged.

The First-hand Experiences

Schedule these with a PTA or group of parents who are learning together:

1. Have your hearing tested for threshold to pure tones, following the same procedures, as nearly as possible, as those that were used to test your own child. Listen for the range of the pitch of tones. Ask to hear the tones at 20, 40, 60 and 80 decibels above your threshold.

2. Now have the audiologist present each tone to one of your ears at the level it had to be presented so that your child could just respond at his hearing threshold. This will give you some idea of the difference between your hearing level and the hearing level of your child.

3. Using a 1000 Hertz tone, ask your audiologist to establish your *tolerance* level to this frequency. Compare this to your hearing *threshold* level for that frequency. Now, compute your dynamic range for 1000 Hertz (tolerance level − hearing threshold level = dynamic range). Compare your dynamic range to that of your own child.

4. Have an audiologist with a speech audiometer let you listen to running conversational speech presented at about 40 to 50 decibels above your hearing threshold, or at a level that you find comfortable for listening. Now have the speech level reduced to 10 or 15 decibels above your hearing threshold and listen for a while. Think about how hard you would have to concentrate to keep understanding speech at this soft level.

5. Arrange for an audiologist with a speech audiometer and sound filters to let you listen to continuous conversational speech, unfiltered, and at a comfortable listening level. Now have the speech filtered so that you can hear only the lower pitches of the speech spectrum, gradually reducing the size of the spectrum until you can hear nothing. Notice that you might be able to hear the rhythm of speech even though you cannot understand it. Do you see why it is possible for your child to hear speech but not understand it?

6. Now have the speech filtered so that you can hear only the higher pitches of the speech spectrum. Note that you could still understand speech even though it sounded unnatural. Gradually reduce the spectrum until you can hearing nothing. Then listen again to the whole speech spectrum at a comfortable level.

7. Have an ear impression and earmold made for one of your ears so that you can use it to listen to one of your child's hearing aids. When the audiologist is sure the hearing aid is working properly, listen to the sound amplified slightly in a variety of situations so that you will have a "par value" against which to compare the hearing aid every day.

8. With your earmold in place and your child's hearing aid turned down very low, listen to someone talking in a very noisy place and note the difficulty you have in sorting out the speech from background noise. Move closer to the speaker and farther away and see how the *ratio* of the speech and the noise changes.

9. Follow the suggestion in Chapter 1 to have an audiologist deliver steady noise to both your ears while you talk to someone. Notice how you and other parents raise your voices as the noise level is raised so that you can hear yourself talk. When you cannot hear yourself, feel the movement of your lips, tongue and jaw as you talk or read something aloud.

WHAT IS THE SPECIAL PART PARENTS PLAY IN HELPING TEACH SPEECH?

People who are experienced in teaching hearing-impaired children to speak agree that success requires three things: (1) a child who wants to talk and is willing to work at it, (2) parents who encourage and help their child, and (3) a school program that is efficient and diligent. They also believe that all these efforts must be coordinated. Figure 9 translates this belief into areas of activity, and illustrates that there is overlapping of responsibility for the *student*, the *environment,* and the *school program.* Use this figure and check off the areas of concern as you read the following paragraphs.

In Chapter 5 we noted the responsibility of the school program to provide *systematic instruction* based on principles of learning, **[pp. 55–57]** and *individualized instruction* that recognizes and responds to important differences among children. **[pp. 54–55]** A complete school program will also see that speech does not end when the child leaves the classroom, and that there is opportunity to use speech in a *school oral environment* that includes the lunch room, recess, interaction in the hallways, and other situations **[pp. 53–54]** that lead to real oral communication.

Parents and school programs share responsibility for enhancing the *sensory abilities* of young children, especially the ability to use hearing for speech through an auditory monitoring program as described in Chapter 4. **[pp. 44–47]** Vision should not be overlooked, either. The parents should see that their child has eye tests from time to time. Some school programs include regular vision screening for their hearing-impaired children. Ask your school about arranging vision screening. **[pp. 47–50]** *Learning abilities* are influenced both by attitudes of the parents and by the motivating environment of the school. Internal or intrinsic motivation of children who want to learn speech because it is important and useful to them, rather than rewarding to the parents or teachers, is the best motivation.

Parents have the primary responsibility for their child's *physical maturation and growth.* **[pp. 42–44]** This is as important for learning speech as it is for learning anything else. Young children grow and mature at fairly

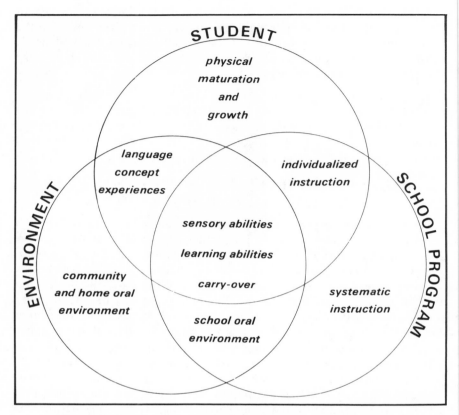

Figure 9. Important areas in learning and teaching speech.

predictable rates. Schedules of progress, based on child development studies, help parents and teachers know what skills of motor coordination can be expected from each child. The jaw grows during early school years, causing spaces between teeth. Abnormalities in physical growth may interfere with speech development.

Language concept experiences are another responsibility of the parents. **[p. 51]** For children to talk, they must have something to say. To have something to say, they must have experiences that lead to ideas that need to be expressed in language. And then they must have opportunities that give them a chance to convey information through speech. Play activities with selected toys, "walking tours" with parents who help discover, examine and name things of interest, and projects shared with parents or siblings, require only the gift of one's time and some common sense. A practical example is creating "experience books." These can be made by parents and children working together as the event is happening, and then are available for refer-

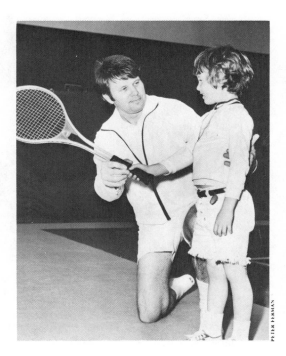

Experiences build language.

ence and review at a later time. Simple "dime-store" spiral notebooks will do. Crayons may be used with younger children where pictures are included, and pen or pencil are fine for older children. Making the experience books during the action ties activities and objects to the appropriate language, and reference at a later time gives opportunity to use spontaneous spoken language about a familiar event.

Carry over from the classroom to the total environment of the student requires cooperation between the school and family that goes well beyond "homework." **[pp. 52–53]** Parents can let the school know about recent experiences of the child so that these can "come up" in language and speech lessons. The school needs to keep parents informed of language recently learned and what to expect in a child's speech. Carry over for teaching speech works best when it is a two-way street. It means not only that parents visit schools, but that teachers sometime visit homes. The result will be an atmosphere of support that the child will not fail to see and appreciate.

We have already suggested some factors in establishing an *"oral environment"* in the *community* and at *home.* This is a very special responsibility of parents. **[p. 52]** Speech is most likely to be learned when it is practiced in an oral environment where its use is constant, consistent, and meaningful.

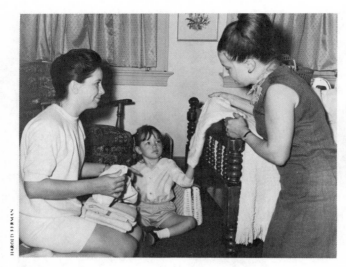

Everyday activities can be language experiences in an oral environment.

These are the important features of an **oral environment:**

1. Speech is the primary *means of communication,* rather than gesturing or manual communication.

2. There should be frequent *need* to use speech. If children are too easily understood when they point or cry, they may continue to do so.

3. There should be a lot of *normal speech* for the child to hear. Don't stop talking to your child. He needs some examples to imitate.

4. There should be many *chances to use* speech. Taking time to listen to a child's comments, no matter how rudimentary, can help the hearing-impaired child understand the usefulness of language.

5. *Encouragement* to use speech. This may have to be through such rewards as candy to begin with, but praise can go a long way toward making a child want to talk. As children grow older, they may need urging in order to succeed and gain confidence for talking in many new situations.

WHERE WILL YOUR CHILD BE ABLE TO USE HIS SPEECH?

The responsive individuals of home and school are generally rewarding to a child, but strangers are another matter. Some people who have never heard hearing-impaired children talk will be so interested in how the child talks that they will not listen to what the child says. Speech is so closely associated with personality that the first time they hear speech from a hearing-impaired child some people will probably be thinking "what's wrong with that child," and feel embarrassed, rather than listening to what the child is saying. *It is natural and human.* What we know from experience is that almost everyone can understand "hearing-impaired speech," given a little time and effort. *The rate of learning to understand the speech of hearing-impaired persons by people with normal hearing is very rapid.* They need to listen and have some success in understanding when the subject of conversation can help them fill in the blanks, and then they gradually get better. Having the child repeat for the listener will help the process.

There are various groups of people in your child's life with whom he will find speech more or less useful. Figure 10 reflects these groups, based on familiarity and amount of contact. **[p. 3]** The expanding circles suggest the expanding opportunities for achievement in society. Some hearing-impaired persons may be limited to one or two of the inner circles. Others will have

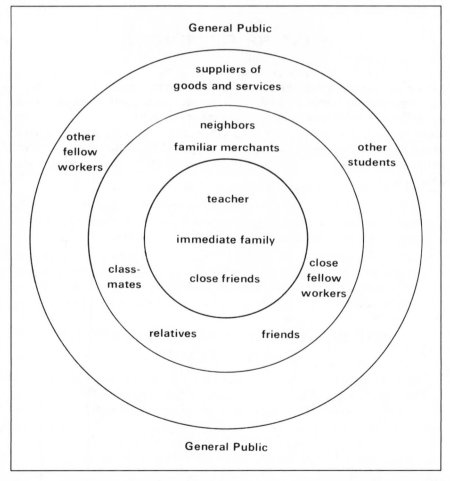

Figure 10. Expanding groups of people with whom speech can be functional.

some limited contacts with the general public, while still others will be unlimited in their scope.

When hearing-impaired children are young, it is likely they will talk mostly to members of the immediate family, teachers and a few close friends. The school should give opportunity to expand this to other children and adult school staff members. But these "inner circles" should not continue to be the only opportunity as a child grows older. Parents may have to take their child in to meet the clerk at a neighborhood store, have the child say a little, perhaps naming things, and then arrange for the child to try a first purchase of a familiar and desired item. This may have to be contrived with the clerk ready for the test, but that may give your child, as well as the clerk, the confidence to try it again. The effort is worthwhile!

WHAT DO YOU DO NOW?

It's time to put this book down and go to work. First you might want to meet with your child's teacher or audiologist and talk over what you can do together for your particular child in your special situation. Keep this book for reference, or share it with other members of your family, friends who come in contact with your child, or classroom teachers. From your own experience you may find some new ideas that will help other parents. Write them down and use them to expand your own *Parents' Guide to Speech and Deafness.*

Suggested Readings

The material listed below may be helpful for families to understand speech and deafness. These publications are available from the Alexander Graham Bell Association for the Deaf, 3417 Volta Place NW, Washington, DC 20007. This is nontechnical material aimed at families rearing hearing-impaired children and those who will be teaching hearing-impaired children without being trained in this field. Your school staff, speech pathologist, or audiologist may suggest some additional reading:

1. Bishop, Milo E. (Ed.). *Mainstreaming: Practical Ideas for Educating Hearing-Impaired Students.* Washington, DC: Alexander Graham Bell Assn. for the Deaf, 1979, 228 pp.

   Based on 10 years experience at the National Technical Institute for the Deaf (NTID), this book is written to help teachers, administrators, and supervisors address the educational needs of hearing-impaired students in the adolescent and young adult age groups. Topics of discussion include individual assessment; practical suggestions for judging whether a student should be mainstreamed; selecting teaching materials; determining how the physical characteristics of the classroom can be varied to assist mainstreaming, and professional and community support services

2. Griffin, Betty F. (Ed.). *Family to Family.* Washington, DC: Alexander Graham Bell Assn. for the Deaf, 1980, 80 pp.

   Ten concerned and articulate parents of hearing-impaired children express their feelings about sixteen topics including speech and language, social and psychological concerns, reading, math and science, health, amplification, independence, physical coordination, resources, projects, and accomplishments.

3. Griffin, Betty F. *My Child Comes with Directions.* Washington, DC: Alexander Graham Bell Assn. for the Deaf, 1978, 32 pp.

   A workbook for parents, advisors, or teachers to record crucial information about the developing hearing-impaired child, covering the child's audiogram, medical history, personal observations, speech and language development, academic development, and hearing aid use.

4. McArthur, Shirley. *Raising your Hearing-Impaired Child: A Guide for Parents.* Washington, DC: Alexander Graham Bell Assn. for the Deaf, 1982, 256 pp.

   A practical and inspiring guidebook that offers much-needed information and support for parents who discover that their child has a hearing loss. The author is the mother of two hearing-impaired children, as well as a teacher of the deaf.

5. Neyhus, Arthur I., & Austin, Gary F. (Eds.). *Deafness and Adolescence.* Washington, DC: Alexander Graham Bell Assn. for the Deaf, 1978, 120 pp.

   A *Volta Review* monograph on all aspects of the hearing-impaired adolescent experience, including psychological and biological development, communication ability, educational needs, and post-secondary curriculum.

6. Northcott, Winifred H. (Ed.). *The Hearing-Impaired Child in a Regular Classroom: Preschool, Elementary, and Secondary Years.* Washington, DC: Alexander Graham Bell Assn. for the Deaf, 1973, 301 pp.

   A practical handbook for teachers, administrators, resources specialists, and parents. Includes over 40 chapters by individuals directly involved in mainstream programs, glossary of terms, and bibliography.

7. Star, Robin R. *We Can!* (Vols. 1 & 2). Washington, DC: Alexander Graham Bell Assn. for the Deaf, 1980, 96 pp. & 104 pp.

   Provides role models for hearing-impaired children. The 31 biographies in this two-volume set profile oral hearing-impaired men and women who have successful careers. These books are written at the 4th-grade level and can be used in the classroom for career education as well as for language and reading instruction.

8. Simmons-Martin, Audrey Ann. *Chats with Johnny's Parents.* Washington DC: Alexander Graham Bell Assn. for the Deaf, 1975, 80 pp.

   An informal discussion of the language learning process, speech-reading, the uses of amplification, auditory training, and speech teaching.

9. Vaughan, Pat. (Ed.). *Learning to Listen.* Washington, DC: Alexander Graham Bell Assn. for the Deaf, 1981, 197 pp.

   A book for parents of young hearing-impaired children. Six mothers relate their experiences in teaching their hearing-impaired children how to listen. The activities, games, and books recommended are excellent for anyone helping a child with a language problem.

Index